The POTS Pregnancy Survival Guide

Evidence-Based Strategies for Managing Symptoms, Navigating Birth, and Optimizing Recovery

Clemence Jemma Scott

ISBN: 978-1-7642720-0-1

Table of Contents

Introduction: Empowering Your Pregnancy Journey

You have Postural Orthostatic Tachycardia Syndrome (POTS). You want to have a baby. And if you've spent more than five minutes online or talked to other patients, you are likely terrified.

The stories are everywhere. People talk about debilitating nausea, fainting in the shower, being unable to work, and the crushing fear that their medication might harm their baby or that *stopping* their medication might make them unable to function. It's easy to fall into the trap of thinking this journey is destined to be a disaster.

Well, I'm here to tell you that thinking is nonsense.

Is pregnancy with POTS hard? Yes, often it is. Does it require meticulous planning, self-discipline, and a willingness to advocate for yourself in a medical system that often doesn't understand your condition? Absolutely. But is it impossible, or must it be a nine-month nightmare? No.

This planner is not going to sugarcoat the realities of managing a complex autonomic disorder while your body undergoes the most significant physiological transformation of its life. But it's also not going to let you wallow in "what-ifs" and anxiety. We are going to deal with reality. We are going to focus on what you can control, optimize your health before you even conceive, and create flexible strategies for the challenges that will inevitably arise.

You are approaching this from a position of strength. You already know how to listen to your body. You already know how to manage symptoms. You are resilient. Now, we're just applying those skills to a new challenge.

Understanding the intersection of POTS pathophysiology and pregnancy hemodynamics

Let's get clear on what's happening in your body. If you don't understand the mechanics, you can't fix the engine.

POTS is, fundamentally, a problem with your autonomic nervous system (ANS). The ANS is your body's automatic control center. It manages the things you don't think about: heart rate, blood pressure, digestion, temperature. In POTS, the biggest failure of this system happens when you stand up.

When a healthy person stands, the ANS tells the blood vessels in the legs and abdomen to tighten up. This prevents gravity from pulling all the blood down to their feet. It ensures enough blood gets back to the heart and then up to the brain.

When *you* stand up, that tightening mechanism doesn't work correctly. Gravity wins. Blood pools in your lower body. Your brain senses this drop in blood flow and panics. It sends a distress signal (often in the form of adrenaline) to your heart, telling it to beat faster to compensate for the low blood return.

This leads to the diagnostic criteria: a sustained heart rate increase of at least 30 beats per minute (bpm) within 10 minutes of standing, without a significant drop in blood pressure (Raj et al., 2022). But the symptoms are what you actually feel: dizziness, brain fog, fatigue, palpitations, nausea, and sometimes fainting (syncope).

Now, let's throw pregnancy into the mix.

Pregnancy is a massive cardiovascular event. It changes everything about how your blood flows. Here are the main changes (Morgan et al., 2022):

1. **Increased Blood Volume:** This is the big one. Your total blood volume increases by 30% to 50%. This starts early in the first trimester and peaks around the 34th week. This extra fluid is necessary to support the placenta and the growing fetus.

2. **Increased Cardiac Output:** Your heart has to work harder to move all that extra fluid. Cardiac output (the amount of blood your heart pumps per minute) increases significantly.

3. **Hormonal Changes and Vasodilation:** Pregnancy hormones, particularly progesterone and estrogen, cause your blood vessels to relax and widen (*vasodilation*). This is meant to accommodate the higher blood volume, but it actually causes maternal blood pressure to decrease, usually hitting its lowest point in the second trimester.

4. **Increased Heart Rate:** Even in healthy pregnancies, the resting heart rate increases by 10 to 20 bpm.

See the conflict?

POTS is often characterized by low effective blood volume and difficulty keeping blood vessels tight. Pregnancy increases blood volume (which should help) but also relaxes blood vessels and increases the baseline heart rate (which can make things worse).

If your POTS is primarily driven by hypovolemia (low blood volume), the massive increase in fluid during pregnancy might make you feel significantly better. The extra fluid fills up those relaxed vessels, improving blood return to the heart.

However, if your POTS has a strong hyperadrenergic component (too much adrenaline/sympathetic drive), or if the vasodilation (relaxed vessels) outweighs the volume increase, your symptoms might explode. The hormonal shifts can exacerbate nausea and fatigue, and the relaxed vessels mean even *more* blood pooling.

Understanding this intersection is power. It explains why your symptoms might change drastically throughout the pregnancy and why one-size-fits-all advice is useless.

Addressing symptom variability (Worsening, improving, and fluctuating)

If you are looking for a guarantee about how you will feel during pregnancy, you won't find one. The course of POTS during pregnancy is highly variable. Stop demanding certainty where none exists. Instead, prepare for variability.

The research reflects this unpredictability, though recent, larger studies suggest a more challenging course for many.

Older, smaller studies often presented a rosier picture. For example, a study of 22 patients found that 55% reported improvement, 31% reported worsening, and 13% reported no change (Kanjwal et al., 2009). This data is often cited to reassure patients.

However, a much larger cross-sectional survey involving over 1,600 pregnancies painted a different picture. This study found that 81.1% of participants experienced symptom worsening at some point during their pregnancy (Dangel et al., 2023).

Let's look at the breakdown from that larger study (Dangel et al., 2023):

- **First Trimester:** 62.6% experienced worsening symptoms.

- **Second Trimester:** 48.2% experienced worsening symptoms (indicating improvement for some compared to the first trimester).

- **Third Trimester:** 58.9% experienced worsening symptoms.

What does this tell us?

First, the first trimester is often the hardest. This is when hormonal shifts are most dramatic, nausea is common, and the blood volume expansion hasn't fully kicked in yet. If you feel terrible in the first trimester, it doesn't mean the whole pregnancy will be that way. The study found that if symptoms improved in the first trimester, that improvement often persisted; but early worsening was common (Dangel et al., 2023).

Second, the second trimester often offers a reprieve. This is the "golden period" for many. Blood volume is high, but the physical burden of the late third trimester hasn't started.

Third, the third trimester gets tough again. The physical size of the uterus can compress major blood vessels (like the vena cava), reducing blood return to the heart, especially when lying down. The increased cardiac demand also adds stress.

And then there's the postpartum period. The sudden drop in blood volume after delivery, combined with sleep deprivation and the physical demands of newborn care, often triggers significant flares. The Dangel et al. (2023) study found that 58.7% reported worse symptoms 3 months postpartum compared to their pre-pregnancy baseline.

Case Example: Sarah's Rollercoaster

Sarah, 29, had moderately severe POTS managed with Midodrine and high salt intake before pregnancy. She was anxious but optimized her health beforehand. The first 14 weeks were brutal. She developed hyperemesis gravidarum (severe vomiting), couldn't keep fluids down, and her POTS symptoms flared dramatically. She required IV fluids at home. She felt defeated.

But around week 16, things shifted. The nausea subsided, and the increased blood volume kicked in. From week 16 to week 30, she felt better than she had in years. She stopped the Midodrine because she didn't need it. She was energetic and optimistic.

At week 32, the fatigue and tachycardia returned. She struggled with shortness of breath and couldn't stand for long periods due to the physical pressure of the late pregnancy. She managed with compression and rest. Her delivery was smooth, but the first month postpartum was extremely difficult as her blood volume dropped and she resumed medication.

Sarah's experience is typical in its *atypicality*. It fluctuated. The key to managing this is not to panic when a flare happens or get complacent when things are good. It's about having the tools ready and adjusting your strategies day by day.

Translating clinical evidence into actionable strategies

You may have noticed that the medical literature on POTS and pregnancy is sparse. There are no large-scale clinical trials and no universal consensus guidelines for management during pregnancy (Morgan et al., 2022). Much of what we know comes from expert opinion, case reports, and retrospective reviews.

Furthermore, the information that *does* exist is often buried in medical journals, written in dense, inaccessible language. You don't have time to become a cardiologist while you're preparing for a baby.

That's the purpose of this planner. We are taking the best available clinical evidence—like the 2021 POTS Expert Consensus Review (Vernino et al., 2021) and recent comprehensive reviews on POTS in pregnancy (Morgan et al., 2022)—and translating it into clear, actionable strategies.

We aren't just telling you *what* to do; we are telling you *why*.

For example:

- **Clinical Evidence:** Increased blood volume is central to managing POTS, and hydration needs increase during pregnancy.

- **Actionable Strategy:** Aim for at least 2.5 liters of fluids and at least 7 grams of salt per day during pregnancy (Morgan et al., 2022). We will provide tools for tracking this and strategies for achieving it even when nauseated.

- **Clinical Evidence:** Venous pooling is exacerbated by prolonged standing and heat.

- **Actionable Strategy:** Utilize waist-high maternity compression garments (20-30 mmHg). Modify daily activities (sit while cooking, use a shower chair). Avoid heat triggers.

- **Clinical Evidence:** Deconditioning worsens POTS symptoms by reducing muscle mass and plasma volume (Fu & Levine, 2018).

- **Actionable Strategy:** Engage in structured, graded exercise focusing on recumbent activities (swimming, rowing, recumbent cycling) and lower body strength training, adapted for the physiological changes of pregnancy.

This planner focuses on proactive management. We are not waiting for a crisis to happen. We are anticipating the challenges and putting preventative measures in place.

How to use this planner: A roadmap for proactive management

This book is structured to follow the timeline of your pregnancy journey, starting where you should ideally begin: 6 to 12 months *before* conception.

Part I: The Foundation (Pre-Conception Optimization)

This is arguably the most important section. The healthier and more stable you are before pregnancy, the better you will handle the stresses ahead. We will cover optimizing your symptoms, reviewing medication safety, nutritional preparation, building your medical team, and preparing your support system. Look, if you fail to plan, you are planning to fail. It's that simple.

Part II: Navigating Pregnancy (Trimester by Trimester)

We will break down the specific challenges of each trimester. This includes managing nausea and fatigue in the first trimester, adapting to blood volume changes in the second, and preparing for delivery in the third. We will provide strategies for hydration, exercise, work accommodations, and symptom tracking.

Part III: Delivery and Birth

Labor and delivery are high-stress hemodynamic events. We will discuss anesthesia considerations (epidurals can cause blood pressure drops), optimal positioning, fluid management during labor, and specific considerations for Cesarean births. The goal is a safe delivery with minimal autonomic chaos.

Part IV: The Fourth Trimester and Beyond (Recovery and Parenthood)

The immediate postpartum period is often when POTS patients struggle the most. We will address the postpartum hemodynamic shift, breastfeeding challenges, medication resumption, sleep deprivation, and the mental health challenges of new parenthood with a chronic illness.

Part V: The POTS Pregnancy Toolkit

This section provides concrete tools: checklists, communication scripts, birth plan templates, symptom logs, and organizers. You should photocopy these, fill them out, and use them actively.

A Note on Mindset:

As you use this planner, you must actively fight against the urge to catastrophize. It is rational to be concerned about potential complications. It is irrational to assume they *will* happen and that you won't be able to handle them.

Pregnancy with POTS requires flexibility, resilience, and a commitment to the strategies outlined here. You can do this. It won't be perfect, but it can be successful.

Chapter 1: Preparing Your Body and Mind

If you are already pregnant and reading this, don't panic. Start applying these principles today. But if you are planning ahead—which is the smart thing to do—you should give yourself 6 to 12 months before trying to conceive.

Why so long? Because optimizing your health with POTS is not a quick fix. It takes time to adjust medications, implement a sustainable exercise routine, correct nutritional deficiencies, and stabilize your symptoms. Pregnancy is a marathon, and you wouldn't show up to a marathon without training.

This pre-conception period is about building your physiological reserves. You want to be as strong, stable, and healthy as possible before your body diverts its resources to growing a human. This chapter is about the rigorous, sometimes frustrating, but absolutely necessary work of getting your house in order.

Achieving baseline symptom stability: Defining "optimized" health

What does it mean to have "optimized" health with POTS? Let's be clear: it does not mean cured. It does not mean symptom-free. If you are waiting for a day when you feel like a "normal" person before getting pregnant, you might be waiting forever. Stop demanding perfection.

Optimized health means your symptoms are managed to the point where you can consistently perform your activities of daily living, maintain adequate nutrition and hydration, and engage in regular physical activity. It means you are not in a constant state of flare or crisis.

Here's a checklist to define your baseline stability:

- **Hydration and Nutrition:** You can consistently consume your target fluid and salt intake daily without significant gastrointestinal distress.

- **Symptom Management:** Dizziness and pre-syncope (feeling like you are about to faint) are manageable and infrequent. Tachycardia is controlled with your current treatment plan (lifestyle and/or medication).

- **Activity Level:** You can tolerate a baseline level of physical activity (e.g., 20-30 minutes of recumbent exercise several times a week) without triggering severe post-exertional malaise (a crash after activity).

- **Comorbid Conditions:** Any co-existing conditions (like MCAS, EDS, migraine, GI issues) are also stable and managed.

If you are currently bedbound, struggling with daily fainting, or unable to tolerate food and fluids, now is not the time to get pregnant. Your priority must be working with your POTS specialist to improve your baseline function.

The Role of Pacing and Energy Management

Achieving stability often requires a rigorous commitment to *pacing*. Pacing means balancing activity with rest to avoid the boom-bust cycle (overdoing it on a good day and then crashing for several days).

You need to understand your *energy envelope*. This is the amount of energy you have available on any given day. If you exceed it, you pay for it later. During the pre-conception phase, your goal is to gradually expand that envelope through exercise and lifestyle management, but also to respect its limits.

If you are constantly pushing yourself to the point of exhaustion because you feel you "should" be doing more, you are sabotaging your stability. Be realistic about what you can do. It is better to do a little bit consistently than to do a lot inconsistently.

Medication review and adjustments: Safety profiles and weighing risks vs. benefits

This is often the biggest source of anxiety for women with POTS planning pregnancy. Medications that help you function might pose risks to a developing fetus. But stopping medications might cause your health to deteriorate, which is also risky for a pregnancy.

There's a crucial reality you must accept: **There are no risk-free choices here.**

Every decision is a balance between maternal health and fetal safety. This requires open, honest conversations with your POTS specialist and a high-risk obstetrician (Maternal-Fetal Medicine or MFM).

The goal of the pre-conception period is to find the safest, most effective medication regimen for pregnancy. This might mean switching medications, adjusting dosages, or intensifying non-pharmacological treatments to reduce reliance on drugs. This process can take months, as tapering off one medication and starting another often causes temporary flares.

General Principles for Medication in Pregnancy:

1. **Lowest Effective Dose:** Use the smallest dose necessary to maintain stability.

2. **Minimize Exposure:** If possible, and only if maternal health allows, medications might be reduced during the critical first trimester (organ development). However, this is often when POTS symptoms are worst.

3. **Data Limitations:** We have limited data on the use of many POTS medications in pregnancy. Most fall into Category C (risks cannot be ruled out, but benefits may outweigh risks).

Let's review the common POTS medications (Morgan et al., 2022; Vernino et al., 2021):

Beta-Blockers (e.g., Propranolol, Metoprolol)

- **Function:** Slow the heart rate and reduce the impact of adrenaline.

- **Pregnancy Safety:** Generally considered relatively safe. Propranolol and Labetalol have been used extensively in pregnancy for conditions like high blood pressure.

- **Potential Risks:** There is some concern that beta-blockers may be associated with fetal growth restriction (small babies), low blood sugar in the newborn, and slow heart rate in the newborn.

- **Strategy:** If necessary for symptom control, they are often continued. Low-dose Propranolol (e.g., 5 mg twice daily) or Metoprolol are often preferred (Morgan et al., 2022). The fetus will need monitoring for growth.

Midodrine

- **Function:** Tightens blood vessels (vasoconstriction) to improve blood return to the heart and raise blood pressure.

- **Pregnancy Safety:** Limited data. It is a Category C drug.

- **Potential Risks:** Because it constricts blood vessels, there is a theoretical concern that it could reduce blood flow to the placenta. However, existing case reports have not shown harmful effects on fetal development (POTS UK, 2021).

- **Strategy:** Often continued if necessary for the mother to remain upright and functional. It should be used only if other measures fail to control symptoms adequately. A typical pregnancy dose might be 2.5-5 mg three times daily (Morgan et al., 2022).

Fludrocortisone (Florinef)

- **Function:** Helps the kidneys retain sodium and water, thereby increasing blood volume.

- **Pregnancy Safety:** Generally considered safe. It has been used for many years in pregnant women with Addison's disease without documented adverse effects (POTS UK, 2021).

- **Potential Risks:** Can cause fluid retention and high blood pressure if not monitored. Requires monitoring of potassium levels.

- **Strategy:** Often continued, especially in patients with hypovolemic POTS. Doses are typically 0.05-0.1 mg daily.

Ivabradine (Corlanor)

- **Function:** Slows the heart rate through a different mechanism than beta-blockers, without affecting blood pressure.

- **Pregnancy Safety: Contraindicated.**

- **Potential Risks:** Animal studies have shown evidence of fetal toxicity and birth defects (teratogenicity).

- **Strategy:** Ivabradine must be discontinued before conception. Women taking it must use reliable contraception. If you are on Ivabradine, the pre-conception period is essential for transitioning to a safer alternative (like a beta-blocker) and ensuring stability.

Pyridostigmine (Mestinon)

- **Function:** Enhances communication between nerves and muscles, which can help stabilize autonomic function.

- **Pregnancy Safety:** Considered relatively safe (Category B). It has been used safely for decades in pregnant women with myasthenia gravis.

- **Strategy:** May be a good option if symptoms worsen during pregnancy, often at a dose of 30 mg twice daily (Morgan et al., 2022).

Stimulants (e.g., Adderall, Ritalin)

- **Function:** Used by some POTS patients to manage brain fog and fatigue, and can also increase vasoconstriction.

- **Pregnancy Safety:** Generally recommended to avoid during pregnancy.

- **Strategy:** Should be tapered and discontinued before conception if possible.

Case Example: Maria's Medication Transition

Maria, 32, relied heavily on Ivabradine (7.5mg twice daily) and occasional stimulants for her POTS. When she decided she wanted to get pregnant, she met with her cardiologist and MFM specialist. They agreed the Ivabradine and stimulants had to go.

The transition was rough. They started by slowly reducing the Ivabradine while introducing low-dose Propranolol. Maria's heart rate increased, and her energy plummeted. She had to take a temporary leave from work. They intensified her salt and fluid intake and focused heavily on her exercise program. It took four months, but she eventually stabilized on Propranolol 10mg twice daily. She found that while her heart rate control wasn't quite as good as with Ivabradine, it was manageable. The stimulants were easier to stop, but she had to accept a lower baseline energy level.

By planning ahead, Maria avoided the risk of Ivabradine exposure to the fetus and ensured she was stable on a safer regimen before conceiving.

The Bottom Line on Meds:

Stop agonizing over the "perfect" choice. Make the most rational choice based on the available data and your specific clinical situation. The risk of uncontrolled maternal POTS—leading to falls, malnutrition, dehydration, and inability to care for yourself—is often greater than the risk of medications like beta-blockers or fludrocortisone.

Nutritional optimization: Salt, fluids, and managing deficiencies

Nutrition in POTS is not just about "eating healthy." It's a primary treatment modality. During pre-conception, you need to optimize your intake of the elements that support autonomic function and ensure you have the necessary reserves for pregnancy.

Salt (Sodium Chloride)

Salt is crucial for POTS patients because it helps the body hold onto water, which increases blood volume. If your blood volume is higher, your heart doesn't have to work as hard when you stand up.

- **Target Intake:** The general recommendation for POTS is 3-10 grams of sodium per day (Vernino et al., 2021). During pregnancy, experts recommend at least 7 grams of salt (sodium chloride) per day (Morgan et al., 2022). (Note: 1 teaspoon of table salt contains about 2.3 grams of sodium).

- **Strategy:** Don't just rely on salty snacks. Integrate salt into your meals. Use salt tablets or high-quality electrolyte powders if you struggle to get enough from food. It's important to build this habit *before* pregnancy, especially before first-trimester nausea makes high salt intake difficult.

Fluids

Fluid intake must accompany high salt intake. If you eat a lot of salt without enough water, you will just get dehydrated.

- **Target Intake:** Generally 2-3 liters per day. During pregnancy, the recommendation increases to at least 2.5 liters (Morgan et al., 2022).

- **Strategy:** Carry a water bottle everywhere. Set timers if you forget. Drink a large glass of water before you even get out of bed in the morning to boost your volume before standing.

Managing Deficiencies

POTS patients are prone to certain nutritional deficiencies, often due to co-existing gastrointestinal issues or restricted diets. Pregnancy increases the demand for specific nutrients. Pre-conception is the time to test for and correct these.

- **Iron:** Iron deficiency (anemia) is common in women of childbearing age and is exacerbated during pregnancy due to increased blood volume. Iron deficiency worsens POTS symptoms like fatigue and tachycardia. Get your ferritin levels checked (this is your iron stores, not just your hemoglobin). If low, start supplementation under medical supervision.

- **Vitamin D:** Crucial for bone health and immune function. Deficiency is common. Test and supplement as needed.

- **Folate (Folic Acid):** Essential for preventing neural tube defects in the fetus. All women planning pregnancy should take a prenatal vitamin containing adequate folate (at least 400 mcg) starting at least 1-3 months before conception.

- **B Vitamins (especially B12):** Important for energy production and nerve function. Deficiency can mimic or worsen POTS symptoms.

Dietary Approaches

While there is no single "POTS diet," certain approaches can help stabilize symptoms:

- **Small, Frequent Meals:** Large, heavy meals divert blood to the digestive system, which can worsen orthostatic intolerance. Eating smaller meals throughout the day can help maintain stable energy and blood sugar levels.

- **Lower Carbohydrate Intake:** High-carb meals, especially refined sugars, can also cause blood pooling in the gut and trigger symptom flares in some patients. Focus on balanced meals with protein, healthy fats, and complex carbohydrates.

- **Gluten-Free:** Some evidence suggests a higher prevalence of Celiac disease and gluten intolerance in POTS patients. A trial of a gluten-free diet may be worthwhile if you have significant GI symptoms (Zha et al., 2022).

The goal here is consistency. Find a nutritional strategy that works for your body and stick to it. Don't jump on every new diet trend. Focus on the fundamentals: salt, fluids, and nutrient density.

Physical conditioning: Graded exercise protocols (e.g., Levine/CHOP) and pelvic floor preparation

If you take only one piece of advice from this chapter, let it be this: **You must exercise.**

I know what you're thinking. "But exercise makes me feel worse!" "I'm too tired to exercise." "My heart rate goes too high."

These are excuses. And they are excuses that will guarantee a more difficult pregnancy.

Exercise is the most effective long-term treatment for POTS (Fu & Levine, 2018). It increases blood volume, strengthens the heart muscle (improving stroke volume), improves the muscle pump in the legs (which helps return blood to the heart), and helps retrain the autonomic nervous system.

If you are deconditioned before pregnancy, the increased cardiovascular demands of pregnancy will hit you much harder.

However, the *way* you exercise matters. You cannot just jump on a treadmill and hope for the best. You need a structured, graded protocol designed for POTS patients.

The Levine Protocol and CHOP Modification

The most well-studied approach is the Levine Protocol, developed by Dr. Benjamin Levine. A common adaptation used in many centers is the CHOP (Children's Hospital of Philadelphia) Modified Dallas POTS Exercise Program.

These protocols share key principles:

1. **Gradual Progression:** They start very slowly and gradually increase the duration and intensity over several months.

2. **Recumbent Exercise First:** Critically, the initial phase focuses on horizontal or seated exercises. This allows you to condition your cardiovascular system without triggering severe orthostatic stress.

   o   Examples: Recumbent bike, rowing machine, swimming (excellent because the water pressure supports circulation).

3. **Transition to Upright:** Only after several months of consistent recumbent exercise do you gradually introduce upright activities (like the elliptical or walking).

4. **Strength Training:** Includes lower body and core strengthening exercises to improve the muscle pump.

5. **Heart Rate Monitoring:** Workouts are often guided by specific heart rate zones to ensure you are working hard enough to achieve conditioning but not so hard that you trigger a severe flare.

Implementing the Protocol

You can find the CHOP protocol online (Dysautonomia International, n.d.). It is typically a 5-7 month program. This is why the 6-12 month pre-conception window is so important. You need time to complete the program and establish a maintenance routine.

Yes, it is hard. Especially in the beginning. You might feel worse before you feel better. You must push through this initial phase, adhering strictly to the protocol. Consistency is more important than intensity.

If you have severe exercise intolerance or co-existing conditions like Myalgic Encephalomyelitis/Chronic Fatigue Syndrome (ME/CFS), you may need a more individualized approach, potentially working with a physical therapist experienced in POTS. But immobilization and bed rest will only make things worse in the long run.

Pelvic Floor Preparation

The pelvic floor is a group of muscles that support the pelvic organs (bladder, uterus, rectum). Pregnancy and childbirth put significant strain on these muscles. POTS patients, especially those with co-existing hypermobility (like EDS), may already have pelvic floor dysfunction.

Pre-conception is the ideal time to start pelvic floor physical therapy. A specialized physical therapist can assess your pelvic floor strength and function and teach you exercises (like Kegels, but often more nuanced) to both strengthen and relax these muscles.

A healthy pelvic floor can help prevent issues like incontinence and pelvic pain during pregnancy and improve postpartum recovery. Don't neglect this. It's foundational strength that you will desperately need.

Mental health preparation: Establishing therapeutic support and coping strategies

Let's talk about your anxiety. It's high, isn't it? You are worried about the pregnancy, the medications, the delivery, and whether you will be able to care for a newborn while managing a chronic illness.

These are valid concerns. But when valid concern tips over into constant rumination, catastrophizing, and panic, it becomes a major problem. Anxiety is not just a mental state; it has physiological consequences. It activates the sympathetic nervous system (the fight-or-flight response), which can directly worsen POTS symptoms like tachycardia and hyperadrenergic flares.

If you don't get a handle on your anxiety before pregnancy, it will likely escalate. The risk of Perinatal Mood and Anxiety Disorders (PMADs) is higher in women with chronic illnesses.

Pre-conception is the time to build your mental health toolkit.

Establishing Therapeutic Support

If you are not already seeing a therapist, find one now. Specifically, look for a therapist who has experience with chronic illness and utilizes evidence-based approaches like Cognitive Behavioral Therapy (CBT) or Acceptance and Commitment Therapy (ACT).

- **CBT** helps you identify and challenge irrational thought patterns (like catastrophizing). For example, changing "I will definitely faint during labor and it will be a disaster" to "I am concerned about managing my symptoms during labor, so I am creating a plan with my medical team."

- **ACT** focuses on accepting the difficult physical sensations and emotions that come with POTS, while committing to actions that align with your values (like becoming a parent).

Therapy is not about complaining. It's about developing concrete skills to manage the psychological burden of POTS and pregnancy.

Developing Coping Strategies

You need practical tools to manage anxiety and stress in the moment.

- **Mindfulness and Grounding:** While mindfulness won't cure POTS, it can help regulate the nervous system's response to symptoms. Grounding techniques can help when you feel panicky or dissociated due to high adrenaline.

22

- **Physiological Sigh:** Deep breathing exercises can sometimes worsen dizziness in POTS patients. A technique called the *physiological sigh* (two quick inhales followed by a long, slow exhale) can be more effective at calming the nervous system.

- **Realistic Expectations:** Much of your stress likely comes from demanding that you feel good all the time. You won't. Accept that some days will be hard. Stop fighting reality. Focus on functioning despite the discomfort.

Addressing Medical PTSD

Many POTS patients have experienced medical gaslighting, dismissal, or traumatic medical events before getting diagnosed. This history can make interacting with the medical system during pregnancy extremely stressful. You might be hyper-vigilant, distrustful of providers, or terrified of procedures.

If you have medical PTSD, it is crucial to address it in therapy before pregnancy. You need to be able to communicate effectively and calmly with your obstetric team, even when you are scared.

Preparing your body and mind for pregnancy is a significant undertaking. It requires discipline, planning, and a willingness to face uncomfortable realities. But this upfront investment will pay dividends. By achieving baseline stability, optimizing your treatment plan, and strengthening your physical and mental resilience, you are giving yourself the best possible chance for a healthy and successful pregnancy

Optimizing Your Pregnancy Foundation

- **Define stability realistically.** Optimized health with POTS does not mean being symptom-free. It means being able to consistently manage daily activities, hydration, and physical activity without constant crises. If you are severely debilitated, prioritize stabilizing your health before attempting conception.

- **Review medications 6-12 months prior.** Every medication choice involves balancing maternal health and fetal safety. Work with your specialists to transition to the safest effective regimen. Beta-blockers, Fludrocortisone, and Pyridostigmine are generally considered relatively safe. Ivabradine is contraindicated and must be stopped before conception.

- **Treat nutrition as medicine.** Establish habits of high salt intake (aiming for 7+ grams/day in pregnancy) and high fluid intake (aiming for 2.5+ liters/day) before conception. Correct deficiencies in iron, Vitamin D, and B12, and ensure you are taking a prenatal vitamin with folate.

- **Commit to graded exercise.** Exercise is non-negotiable. It is the most effective long-term treatment for POTS and crucial for preparing your cardiovascular system for pregnancy. Utilize structured protocols like the Levine or CHOP program, starting with recumbent exercises and gradually progressing.

- **Prioritize mental resilience.** Anxiety and stress directly worsen POTS symptoms. Establish support with a therapist experienced in chronic illness (using CBT or ACT) before pregnancy. Develop coping strategies and address any history of medical trauma.

Chapter 2: Assembling Your Team and Resources

You cannot manage a POTS pregnancy alone. And frankly, you shouldn't try. This isn't a situation where you can just show up at your local OB/GYN and hope for the best. You need a specialized team. You need coordinated care. And you need to be the active manager of that team.

If you try to navigate this with a standard OB who doesn't understand autonomic dysfunction, you are setting yourself up for frustration, anxiety, and potentially unsafe outcomes. You need experts. And you need them lined up *before* you conceive. This chapter is about how to find the right people, how to communicate effectively with them, and how to ensure all aspects of your health—including comorbidities—are addressed.

Building the ideal medical team (High-Risk OB/Maternal-Fetal Medicine (MFM), POTS specialist (Cardiology/Neurology), Anesthesia consultation)

Your team needs to be multidisciplinary. This means doctors from different specialties working together. You are the captain of this team. Your job is to make sure everyone is talking to each other.

Here are the key players you need on your roster:

1. Maternal-Fetal Medicine (MFM) or High-Risk Obstetrician

Let's be clear: A standard OB-GYN is usually not sufficient for a POTS pregnancy. You need a Maternal-Fetal Medicine (MFM) specialist. These doctors have extra training in managing pregnancies complicated by chronic medical conditions.

POTS automatically classifies your pregnancy as high-risk. Don't let that term scare you. It's just a classification that ensures you get the appropriate level of monitoring and care. It means people are paying closer attention.

Finding the Right MFM: This is crucial and sometimes difficult. You need someone who either has experience with POTS or, at the very least, is willing to listen, learn, and collaborate with your specialists. When interviewing potential MFMs, ask direct questions:

- "What is your experience managing patients with autonomic dysfunction or POTS?"

- "How do you approach fluid management and hemodynamic instability during labor?"

- "Are you comfortable coordinating care closely with my cardiologist/neurologist?"

Listen to their answers carefully. If a doctor dismisses your concerns, seems rushed, or tells you POTS is "just anxiety," walk away. Seriously. You need a partner, not an adversary. You do not have time to waste trying to convince a doctor that your illness is real.

2. POTS Specialist (Cardiology/Neurology)

This is the doctor who currently manages your POTS—usually a cardiologist, neurologist, or electrophysiologist. They will be responsible for medication adjustments before and during pregnancy, managing flares, and providing expertise on your autonomic function.

Your POTS specialist needs to be willing to actively co-manage your care with the MFM. Before conception, ask them to write a detailed letter summarizing your diagnosis, current medications, symptom severity, and specific recommendations for pregnancy and delivery management. This letter is gold. Carry it with you everywhere.

3. Anesthesia Consultation

This is a critical step that many people miss. You absolutely must have an anesthesia consultation well before delivery, ideally before pregnancy or early in the first trimester.

Why? Because anesthesia, particularly epidurals and spinal blocks, causes vasodilation (widening of blood vessels). This can lead to a significant drop in blood pressure. For someone with POTS, this drop can be rapid, severe, and dangerous.

Schedule a consultation with the anesthesia department at the hospital where you plan to deliver. During this consultation, discuss:

- Your specific type of POTS (e.g., hypovolemic, hyperadrenergic).

- Your history of blood pressure instability or reactions to medications.

- The plan for IV fluid loading *before* anesthesia administration. This is essential to prevent hypotension.

- Which vasopressors (medications to raise blood pressure) are preferred if hypotension occurs (e.g., phenylephrine is often favored) (Morgan et al., 2022).

Having an anesthesia plan documented in your chart beforehand is essential for a safe delivery. It prevents scrambling and ensures the team knows exactly what to do.

4. Other Key Players

- **Physical Therapist (PT):** Specifically, one trained in POTS exercise protocols and a pelvic floor specialist.

- **Mental Health Professional:** As discussed in Chapter 1.

- **Other Specialists:** Depending on your comorbidities (e.g., Immunologist for MCAS, Rheumatologist or Geneticist for EDS).

Building this team takes effort. It might require traveling to a larger medical center. It might require making a lot of phone calls. But it is an investment in your safety and the safety of your baby.

Strategies for effective communication and self-advocacy in medical settings

You have your team. Now you have to manage them. Given the lack of widespread knowledge about POTS, you will inevitably encounter healthcare providers—nurses, residents, even attending physicians—who do not understand your condition. They might mistake your symptoms for anxiety or "normal" pregnancy complaints.

You must be prepared to advocate for yourself. Self-advocacy is not about being difficult, aggressive, or demanding. It is about ensuring you receive safe and appropriate care by communicating your needs clearly and effectively.

Here's how to do it rationally and effectively:

1. Be Organized and Evidence-Based

Keep a medical binder. Yes, an actual physical binder. In this digital age, having everything in one place is still incredibly helpful. This binder should include:

- The summary letter from your POTS specialist.

- Your current medication list and dosages, including allergies.

- A brief (one-page) summary of POTS and how it affects *you* personally (your triggers, your main symptoms).

- Key research articles or clinical guidelines relevant to your care (like the Morgan et al., 2022 review on POTS and pregnancy).

When you go to appointments, bring this binder. Do not assume doctors have read your chart or talked to each other. They often haven't.

2. Communicate Concisely and Objectively

Doctors are busy. They have limited time and attention. They respond best to clear, objective data.

Instead of saying: "I feel awful and dizzy all the time."

Say: "My orthostatic intolerance has increased. My heart rate is reaching 140 upon standing, and I am experiencing pre-syncope three times a day. I am adhering to my fluid and salt intake goals."

See the difference? One is a complaint; the other is data. Data drives action.

3. Use "I" Statements and Ask Clarifying Questions

If you disagree with a recommendation or feel unheard, frame it as a question or a statement about your own experience, rather than an accusation. Avoid saying "You are wrong."

- "I am concerned about taking this medication because of my history of adverse reactions. What are the alternatives?"

- "Can you explain the reasoning behind that recommendation? I want to make sure I understand the risks and benefits."

- "My POTS specialist has recommended this specific protocol for hydration. Can we discuss how to implement it here?"

4. Bring a Support Person

Brain fog and fatigue are real. They can make communication difficult, especially during stressful appointments or when you are feeling very sick. Bring your partner, a family member, or a friend who understands your condition.

Before the appointment, discuss your goals and concerns with them. They can take notes, ask questions you might forget, and advocate on your behalf if you are struggling to communicate.

5. Address Dismissal Directly (But Rationally)

It will happen. A provider will dismiss your symptoms or tell you it's "just anxiety." You need to address it calmly and directly. Do not get emotional, even though it is frustrating.

"I understand that anxiety can contribute to symptoms, but I have a diagnosed autonomic disorder. My symptoms are physiological. I need us to focus on the medical management of my POTS."

If a provider continues to be dismissive or refuses to collaborate, it's time to find a new provider. You do not have the energy to waste arguing with people who refuse to listen.

Case Example: Advocating During a Flare

Jenna was 20 weeks pregnant and went to the emergency room with severe vomiting and dehydration. The ER doctor wanted to give her a medication known to worsen tachycardia. Jenna, despite feeling terrible, calmly explained, "I have POTS. That medication can exacerbate my condition. My MFM recommends IV saline and Zofran. Can you please check my chart or call my MFM?" The doctor was initially resistant, brushing her off. Jenna's husband stepped in, showing the doctor the letter from her specialist and firmly repeating the request. The doctor eventually followed the recommended protocol. Jenna's preparedness and her husband's support prevented a potentially dangerous situation.

Managing comorbidities in pre-conception (EDS, MCAS, Migraine)

POTS rarely occurs in isolation. It often travels with friends. Many patients have comorbidities that significantly impact pregnancy planning. The most common are Ehlers-Danlos Syndrome (EDS), Mast Cell Activation Syndrome (MCAS), and migraine. These must be addressed and stabilized before conception. If these are flaring, your pregnancy will be much harder.

Ehlers-Danlos Syndrome (EDS) and Hypermobility Spectrum Disorders (HSD)

EDS is a group of genetic connective tissue disorders. The hypermobile type (hEDS) is frequently seen with POTS. Connective tissue laxity affects not only the joints but also blood vessels and internal organs.

Pregnancy considerations with EDS/HSD (Morgan et al., 2022):

- **Increased Joint Pain and Instability:** The hormone relaxin, which loosens ligaments during pregnancy to prepare for birth, can exacerbate hypermobility. This leads to increased pain and instability, especially in the pelvis (SI joint pain) and back. Physical therapy and supportive garments (like SI belts) are essential.

- **Cervical Insufficiency:** Weakness of the cervix may increase the risk of preterm birth. Your MFM may recommend closer monitoring of cervical length via ultrasound.

- **Tissue Fragility:** There may be an increased risk of preterm rupture of membranes (water breaking early) and potentially postpartum hemorrhage. Wound healing (e.g., after a C-section or tear) may also be impaired.

- **Anesthesia Considerations:** Patients with EDS may respond differently to local anesthetics (like lidocaine) and may be more prone to significant hypotension with epidurals. This must be discussed during the anesthesia consult.

Mast Cell Activation Syndrome (MCAS)

MCAS involves the inappropriate release of chemicals (like histamine) from mast cells, leading to allergic-type symptoms, inflammation, flushing, GI issues, and autonomic instability. The triad of POTS, EDS, and MCAS is increasingly recognized.

Pregnancy considerations with MCAS:

- **Symptom Variability:** Hormonal shifts (especially estrogen) can significantly impact mast cell stability. Some women improve; others worsen dramatically.

- **Medication Safety:** Many first-line MCAS treatments (like H1 and H2 antihistamines such as Zyrtec and Pepcid) are generally considered safe during pregnancy, but this must be confirmed with your immunologist and MFM. Mast cell stabilizers (like Cromolyn Sodium) also generally have a good safety profile.

- **Trigger Avoidance:** Meticulous avoidance of triggers (foods, chemicals, stress, heat) is crucial.

- **Delivery Planning:** A plan must be in place to manage potential allergic reactions or mast cell degranulation during the stress of labor and delivery. This includes awareness of any sensitivities to medications, IV fluids, or surgical materials.

Migraine

Migraine is extremely common in POTS patients. While many women experience improvement in migraines during pregnancy due to stable estrogen levels, others may find they persist or worsen.

Pregnancy considerations with Migraine:

- **Medication Restrictions:** Many common migraine medications (like triptans and some preventative drugs) are restricted or contraindicated during pregnancy.

- **Alternative Treatments:** Focus shifts to non-pharmacological treatments (hydration, trigger avoidance, magnesium supplements, nerve blocks) and potentially safer medications (like certain beta-blockers that treat both POTS and migraine).

- **Preeclampsia Risk:** A history of migraine is associated with a slightly increased risk of hypertensive disorders like preeclampsia, requiring close monitoring of blood pressure (Morgan et al., 2022).

The goal is to have a clear management plan for each comorbidity, coordinated between the relevant specialist and your MFM, before you conceive. Stop ignoring these issues. They matter.

Genetic counseling considerations (especially with EDS)

When you have a chronic illness, it is natural—and rational—to worry about passing it on to your child. This is a heavy emotional burden that needs to be addressed.

POTS Genetics:

POTS does appear to have a familial component, meaning it often runs in families. If you have POTS, your child has a higher chance of developing it than the general population. However, the exact genetic basis is still unclear, and the inheritance pattern is complex. It is likely influenced by multiple genes and environmental factors (e.g., a viral infection might trigger POTS in someone genetically predisposed). Having POTS does not guarantee your child will have it.

EDS Genetics:

The genetics of Ehlers-Danlos Syndrome are more clearly defined. Most types of EDS, including the common hypermobile type (hEDS), are inherited in an *autosomal dominant* pattern. This means if you have EDS, there is a **50% chance** of passing the gene on to your child in each pregnancy.

The Role of Genetic Counseling

If you have a confirmed diagnosis of EDS, or a strong family history of EDS or POTS, meeting with a *genetic counselor* before conception is highly recommended.

A genetic counselor is a professional trained to help you understand genetic risks and make informed decisions. They can help you:

- **Confirm the Diagnosis and Type:** They can help clarify the specific type of EDS. This is very important, as some rare types (like Vascular EDS or vEDS) carry much higher risks in pregnancy, including the risk of arterial rupture. (Note: The specific gene for hEDS has not yet been identified, so diagnosis is clinical, but ruling out other types is crucial).

- **Understand Inheritance Risks:** They can explain the 50% risk and what that means for your family planning.

- **Discuss Options:** They can discuss the available options, which may include prenatal testing (if the specific gene is known) or simply preparing for the possibility of having a child with the condition.

The Emotional Reality

This conversation is hard. You might feel guilt or grief about the possibility of passing on a condition that causes you pain or disability. It is important to process these feelings with your partner and a therapist.

Genetic counseling is not about telling you whether or not to have children. It is about providing you with accurate information so you can make informed decisions that align with your values.

Assembling your resources—your medical team, your knowledge base, and your understanding of your comorbidities and genetics— is a critical step in the pre-conception process. It shifts you from a passive patient to an active manager of your health.

Building Your Support Structure

- **Assemble an expert team early.** You need a Maternal-Fetal Medicine (MFM) specialist, your POTS specialist, and a pre-delivery anesthesia consultation. Do not settle for providers unfamiliar with autonomic dysfunction.

- **Master self-advocacy.** Be organized, bring data (your medical binder), communicate concisely, and ask clarifying questions. You must be an active participant in your care.

- **Optimize comorbidity management.** Work with specialists to stabilize conditions like EDS, MCAS, and migraine before conception, as they significantly impact pregnancy management and risks.

- **Seek genetic counseling if indicated.** Understand the inheritance patterns of your conditions, particularly EDS, to make informed family planning decisions and ensure you have the correct diagnosis (e.g., ruling out Vascular EDS).

Chapter 3: Partner and Support System Preparation

POTS is not a solo journey, especially not during pregnancy. It affects everyone around you—your partner, your family, your friends. If you try to "power through" on your own, hide your symptoms, or refuse help, you are going to crash. Hard. And you will likely breed resentment and misunderstanding in your relationships.

Your support system wants to help, but they often don't know how. They might not understand what POTS is, why you are so exhausted, or what you need from them. It is your job to prepare them. This chapter is about educating your support network, defining roles, and setting clear expectations.

Educating your support system about POTS and pregnancy impacts

You live with POTS every day. You know the symptoms, the triggers, the management strategies. But the people around you? They probably don't get it. They see you looking fine one minute and collapsing the next. They might think you are being dramatic, lazy, or just overly anxious.

This misunderstanding is dangerous. It leads to inadequate support, inappropriate advice ("Just push through it!"), and isolation. You must educate them. Not just about POTS in general, but specifically about how pregnancy changes the game.

Explaining the "Why" (The Spoon Theory)

Don't just say "I'm tired." Explain *why*. One helpful tool is the *Spoon Theory*, developed by Christine Miserandino. It explains what it's like to live with chronic illness.

Imagine you start each day with a limited number of spoons. Each spoon represents a unit of energy. Every activity costs spoons. Getting out of bed costs a spoon. Showering costs two spoons. Cooking costs three spoons. When you run out of spoons, you are done. You cannot do anything else.

Now, explain that POTS means you start the day with fewer spoons than a healthy person. And pregnancy means everything costs more spoons.

Defining the Symptoms Clearly

Use clear, descriptive language to explain your symptoms.

- **Fatigue:** It's not just being tired. It's a profound, heavy exhaustion, like wearing a lead suit. It's a physiological consequence of poor circulation and autonomic dysfunction.

- **Brain Fog:** It's not just forgetfulness. It's difficulty concentrating, finding words, and processing information. It feels like your brain is stuffed with cotton.

- **Dizziness/Pre-syncope:** It's not just lightheadedness. It's the feeling that you are about to faint, often accompanied by tunnel vision, nausea, and a racing heart.

The Impact of Pregnancy

Explain how pregnancy affects POTS. Share the information from the Introduction about the hemodynamic changes (increased blood volume, vasodilation). Help them understand that your symptoms might fluctuate wildly.

Resources for Education

- **Bring Your Partner to Appointments:** Hearing the information directly from your MFM or POTS specialist can be incredibly validating. It shows them that this is a real medical condition that requires serious management.

- **Share Resources:** Provide them with materials from reputable organizations like Dysautonomia International or POTS UK.

- **Have Honest Conversations:** Talk openly about your limitations, your fears, and your needs. Vulnerability builds connection.

Case Example: David's Learning Curve

Chloe has POTS. When she and her husband David started planning for pregnancy, David was supportive but confused. He kept suggesting she "push herself" more, thinking it would help her build stamina. He didn't understand why she needed to sit down in the shower or why she couldn't stand in line at the grocery store. Chloe got frustrated and defensive.

Finally, Chloe sat David down and explained the physiology of POTS using the Spoon Theory. She brought him to her next cardiology appointment. Hearing the doctor emphasize the need for pacing and energy conservation was a turning point for David. He realized that pushing her was actually making things worse. He stopped advising and started asking, "How many spoons do you have left today? What can I take off your plate?"

Education breeds empathy. Empathy breeds effective support.

Defining support roles and household adjustments

When the extreme fatigue and nausea of pregnancy hit, you will not be able to do everything you used to do. This is a fact. If you insist on maintaining the same level of household duties, you will crash. And you will likely end up resenting your partner.

You need to sit down with your partner and explicitly define roles and responsibilities. This might feel awkward or overly formal, but it is essential to prevent burnout and conflict later. Do this *before* you are in crisis.

The Household Audit

Go through every single household task and determine who will be responsible for it, especially during high-symptom periods (like the first trimester and postpartum). Be realistic.

- **Cooking:** This involves a lot of standing. Can your partner take over meal preparation? Can you utilize meal delivery services or batch cook on good days?

- **Cleaning:** Who will clean the bathrooms, vacuum, and do the laundry? Can you afford a cleaning service, even temporarily? If not, you need to accept that the house will be messier. A clean house is not worth a POTS flare.

- **Shopping:** Standing in lines, walking around large stores, and carrying heavy bags are major triggers. Can your partner do the grocery shopping, or can you use grocery delivery services?

- **Childcare (if you have other children):** Who will handle school drop-offs, bedtime routines, and nighttime care?

- **Emotional Labor:** Who is responsible for managing the household schedule, appointments, and finances? This invisible labor is exhausting.

Practical Household Adjustments

Modify your environment to minimize orthostatic stress and conserve energy.

- **Shower Chair:** Essential. Standing in a hot shower is a major POTS trigger. Get one now.

- **Stools:** Place stools in the kitchen (for cooking and dishes) and bathroom (for brushing teeth and getting dressed).

- **Hydration Stations:** Keep water bottles and electrolytes easily accessible throughout the house (bedside table, couch, kitchen).

- **Minimize Stairs:** If you live in a multi-story home, try to set up a resting area on the main floor to avoid unnecessary trips up and down stairs.

- **Reacher/Grabber Tool:** Useful for picking things up off the floor without bending over, which can trigger dizziness.

These adjustments are not about "giving in" to the illness. They are about being smart and strategic. They are about conserving your precious energy for what matters most: growing a healthy baby and maintaining your own stability.

Emergency protocols and communication strategies

What happens if you faint? What happens if you have severe tachycardia, chest pain, or an adverse reaction to a medication? Your support system needs to know how to respond quickly, calmly, and effectively. Panic helps no one.

Creating an Emergency Protocol

You need a clear, written plan. This should be discussed and practiced.

1. **When to Call 911 (or your country's emergency number):** Define the specific criteria. This is crucial because many POTS symptoms (like tachycardia) are chronic and not necessarily emergencies.

41

- Examples: Loss of consciousness for more than 2 minutes, chest pain, difficulty breathing, injury from a fall, signs of stroke.

2. **What to Tell Emergency Responders:** POTS is not always well understood by paramedics. Your partner needs to be able to explain your condition clearly and concisely: "She has Postural Orthostatic Tachycardia Syndrome, an autonomic nervous system disorder. She is pregnant. She needs IV fluids and cardiac monitoring."

3. **Medical Information Sheet:** Keep a one-page summary of your diagnosis, medications, allergies, doctors' contact information, and emergency contacts easily accessible (e.g., on the refrigerator, in your wallet).

4. **Hospital Preference:** Make sure your partner knows which hospital you prefer to go to (the one where your MFM practices).

Communication Strategies

Daily communication is also crucial. How do you tell your partner you are having a bad day without sounding like you are complaining? How do they offer help without being overbearing or patronizing?

- **The Symptom Scale:** Use a 1-10 scale (or the Spoon Theory) to communicate your symptom severity. "I'm at an 8 today. I need to stay on the couch." This provides a quick, objective measure of how you are feeling and what you are capable of.

- **Code Words:** Develop code words or phrases for specific needs. For example, "I need a rescue" might mean "I am feeling faint and need help getting horizontal and getting hydrated immediately."

- **Regular Check-ins:** Schedule regular check-ins (e.g., weekly "state of the union" meetings) to discuss how things are going, what is working, and what needs to change. This is a time to address issues before they fester.

- **Expressing Needs Clearly:** Instead of saying "I wish you would help more," say "I need you to take over dinner tonight because I am too dizzy to stand." Be specific and direct.

Effective communication prevents misunderstandings, reduces conflict, and ensures you get the support you need when you need it.

Financial planning and insurance navigation

Pregnancy is expensive. A high-risk pregnancy with a chronic illness is even more expensive. You might need extra monitoring (ultrasounds, non-stress tests), specialized consultations, expensive medications, or home health services (like IV fluids).

You also need to consider the potential impact on your income. You might need to reduce your work hours, stop working earlier than planned, or take unpaid leave due to severe symptoms.

Financial stress makes POTS worse. It activates the sympathetic nervous system and increases anxiety. Having a financial plan reduces that stress.

Budgeting for Extra Costs

Sit down with your partner and create a realistic budget that includes:

- **Medical Expenses:** Co-pays, deductibles, and out-of-pocket costs for specialists and procedures. Understand your insurance coverage (see below).

- **Medications and Supplements:** The cost of prenatal vitamins, electrolytes (which can be expensive), and any necessary medications.

- **Support Services:** Cleaning services, meal delivery, childcare, or postpartum doula support.

- **Compression Garments:** Medical-grade maternity compression stockings are expensive and often not covered by insurance.

- **Lost Income:** Plan for the possibility of reduced income during pregnancy or an extended maternity leave.

Navigating Insurance

Understanding your health insurance coverage is crucial and often frustrating.

- **Pre-authorizations:** Find out which services require pre-authorization (e.g., home health services, certain medications).

- **In-Network Specialists:** Ensure your MFM and other specialists are covered by your insurance. If not, understand the out-of-network costs.

- **Appealing Denials:** POTS-related treatments (like IV fluids or physical therapy) are sometimes denied by insurance. Learn the appeals process and be prepared to fight for the coverage you need. Keep meticulous records of your symptoms and your doctors' recommendations. Your doctor's office should have staff who can help with this process.

Disability Benefits and Leave Policies

- **Short-Term Disability:** If your symptoms become severe enough that you cannot work, you may qualify for short-term disability benefits. Research the requirements and application process beforehand.

- **FMLA (Family and Medical Leave Act):** In the US, FMLA provides unpaid, job-protected leave for medical reasons, including pregnancy complications. Understand your rights under FMLA and your employer's specific leave policies.

By addressing these practical realities proactively, you can reduce the stress and uncertainty surrounding the financial aspects of your pregnancy journey. It's about taking control of what you can control.

Preparing Your Village

- **Educate Thoroughly:** Ensure your partner and support system understand the physiology of POTS (use the Spoon Theory) and how pregnancy affects it. Bring your partner to key appointments.

- **Define Roles Explicitly:** Conduct a household audit and assign responsibilities clearly. Modify your home environment (shower chair, stools) to conserve energy.

- **Create Emergency Protocols:** Have a written plan for emergencies, including when to call 911 and what information to provide to emergency responders.

- **Develop Communication Strategies:** Use symptom scales or code words to communicate your needs clearly and efficiently. Schedule regular check-ins.

- **Plan Financially:** Budget for extra medical costs (electrolytes, compression, support services) and potential lost income. Understand your insurance coverage and disability benefits.

Chapter 4: The First Trimester (Weeks 1-12): Hormones, Nausea, and Fatigue

The first trimester is, frankly, often brutal for people with POTS. It's a cruel irony. Just when you find out you are pregnant and want to celebrate, your symptoms often flare significantly. If you look at the research, over 60% of women with POTS report worsening symptoms during the first trimester (Dangel et al., 2023).

Why? The hormonal shifts are intense and rapid, and your body hasn't yet built up the extra blood volume that might help stabilize things later.

The first trimester is about survival. It's about managing the nausea, staying hydrated at all costs, and accepting the need for radical rest. Stop trying to be a hero. Just get through it.

Understanding early hemodynamic changes

Right from the moment of conception, your body starts undergoing massive changes. Hormones like progesterone surge. One of the main effects of progesterone is the relaxation of smooth muscle. This is important for the pregnancy, but it also affects your blood vessels, causing them to relax and widen. This is called *vasodilation*.

As we discussed earlier, wider blood vessels mean more blood pooling in your lower body and potentially lower blood pressure. Your autonomic nervous system, which already struggles to keep your blood vessels tight, has to work even harder to maintain circulation.

Here's the kicker: In the first trimester, the vasodilation happens *before* your blood volume has increased significantly. So, you have a bigger "container" (wider blood vessels) but not enough fluid to fill it.

The result: increased tachycardia, more severe dizziness upon standing, and crushing fatigue.

It is important to understand that this is a normal physiological response to pregnancy, amplified by POTS. You aren't failing. You aren't doing anything wrong. Your body is dealing with a massive hemodynamic shift. Normalizing this experience can help reduce the anxiety associated with the symptom flare. Knowing that it often improves in the second trimester can also help you endure it.

Differentiating morning sickness from POTS-related nausea

Nausea is the hallmark of early pregnancy. But nausea is also a very common symptom of POTS. How do you tell the difference? And more importantly, how do you manage this double whammy?

Morning Sickness:

- Caused by hormonal changes (hCG and estrogen).

- Often triggered by specific smells or foods.

- Typically worse in the morning but can occur at any time of day.

- Usually improves by the second trimester.

POTS-Related Nausea:

- Often occurs when you are upright or after prolonged standing (due to reduced blood flow to the brain and gut— the brain interprets this as a crisis and triggers nausea).

- May be associated with dizziness, tachycardia, and pre-syncope.

- Can be caused by autonomic dysfunction affecting gut motility (slow digestion or gastroparesis).

- Worsened significantly by dehydration and low blood volume.

Often, it's a miserable combination of both. The key is to identify the patterns. If the nausea hits when you stand up and improves when you lie down, it's likely POTS-related. If it hits when you smell coffee, it's likely morning sickness.

Management Strategies:

You need to attack the nausea aggressively. It is not just uncomfortable; it interferes with your ability to hydrate and eat, which are essential for managing POTS.

- **Small, Frequent Meals:** An empty stomach often worsens nausea. Keep crackers by your bed and eat something before you even get up. Aim for small snacks every 2-3 hours.

- **Bland Foods:** Focus on simple carbohydrates (crackers, toast, rice) if that is all you can tolerate. Don't worry about a perfectly balanced diet right now. Calories and fluids are the priority.

- **Ginger and Vitamin B6:** Often recommended for morning sickness and can be helpful. Ginger chews or tea can soothe the stomach. Vitamin B6 supplements (usually 25mg three times a day) are safe and effective for many women.

- **Acupressure Bands:** Wristbands (like Sea-Bands) can help reduce nausea for some people.

- **Aggressive Hydration (see below):** Sometimes, POTS nausea improves significantly with adequate fluids and salt. Dehydration itself causes nausea.

If these strategies are not enough, talk to your MFM about anti-nausea medications. Options like Diclegis (a combination of Vitamin

B6 and an antihistamine) or Zofran (Ondansetron) are often used. Do not just suffer through it.

Hyperemesis Gravidarum (HG): High risk in POTS patients and management strategies

Hyperemesis Gravidarum (HG) is extreme, persistent nausea and vomiting during pregnancy. It is not just bad morning sickness. It is a debilitating condition that leads to dehydration, significant weight loss, and electrolyte imbalances.

Here's a critical point: Research suggests that people with POTS may be at a **higher risk** for developing HG (D'Oria et al., 2023). The connection is not fully understood but may be related to the underlying autonomic dysfunction affecting the GI system.

HG is a serious medical condition that requires aggressive management. If you cannot keep fluids down, you get dehydrated. Dehydration makes POTS much worse, which in turn worsens the nausea and vomiting. It's a vicious cycle that can quickly spiral out of control and lead to hospitalization.

Recognizing HG:

How do you know if it's HG and not just normal morning sickness?

- Vomiting multiple times a day (often more than 3-4 times).

- Inability to keep down food or fluids for 24 hours.

- Significant weight loss (more than 5% of pre-pregnancy weight).

- Signs of dehydration (dark urine, extreme dizziness, dry mouth, rapid heart rate even when lying down).

Management Strategies:

- **Early Intervention:** This is key. Do not wait until you are severely dehydrated to seek help. Contact your MFM immediately if you suspect HG. Be persistent.

- **Medication Escalation:** Stronger anti-nausea medications are essential. You may need a combination of drugs.

- **IV Hydration:** Often necessary to break the cycle of dehydration and vomiting (more on this below).

- **Nutritional Support:** If you are unable to eat, you may need nutritional support, such as specialized drinks or, in severe cases, tube feeding or total parenteral nutrition (TPN), although this is rare.

If you have a history of HG in previous pregnancies, or if you have severe GI issues related to POTS, you need a proactive plan in place before the nausea even starts. Discuss medication options and hydration strategies with your MFM early on.

Fluid and electrolyte adjustments (including IV hydration options when oral intake is difficult)

Staying hydrated is the cornerstone of POTS management. We aim for 2.5-3 liters of fluid and 7+ grams of salt per day. But what happens when you are too nauseous to drink, or when you vomit everything you consume?

You cannot just "power through" dehydration. It is dangerous for you and the baby. You need alternative strategies.

Maximizing Oral Intake:

- **Small Sips:** Don't try to drink large amounts at once. Drink small amounts of fluid frequently throughout the day. Set a timer if you need to.

- **Ice Chips or Popsicles:** Sometimes tolerated better than liquid water. You can make your own electrolyte popsicles.

- **Electrolyte Powders:** Use high-quality, high-sodium electrolyte solutions (like Normalyte, Liquid IV, LMNT). The salt is crucial for retaining the fluid.

- **Cold Fluids:** Often better tolerated than room temperature fluids.

- **Avoid Plain Water:** Drinking too much plain water can flush out your electrolytes, making you feel worse.

The Role of IV Hydration

If oral hydration is not enough, **IV hydration** is a safe and effective option. Getting 1-2 liters of Normal Saline or Lactated Ringer's solution can rapidly replenish your blood volume, reduce POTS symptoms, and often significantly improve nausea.

Many POTS patients require regular IV fluids during the first trimester (e.g., 1-2 times per week) or throughout the pregnancy if HG persists.

Setting up IV Hydration:

Discuss this option with your MFM proactively, before you are in crisis.

- **Infusion Centers:** Your doctor can prescribe IV fluids to be administered at an outpatient infusion center.

- **Home Health Services:** In some areas, home health nurses can administer IV fluids at home. This is often the most comfortable and convenient option, but insurance coverage can be tricky.

- **Emergency Room/Hospital Admission:** If you are severely dehydrated, you may need to go to the ER or be admitted to the hospital for rapid rehydration and monitoring.

Advocacy for IV Fluids:

Some doctors are hesitant to prescribe IV fluids, viewing them as unnecessary or risky. However, in the context of POTS and HG, they are often medically necessary. You may need to advocate for this treatment. Having your POTS specialist communicate the need for aggressive hydration to your MFM can be helpful.

Managing extreme fatigue and brain fog

The fatigue of the first trimester is unlike anything else. It's a profound, cellular exhaustion. Add POTS fatigue on top of that, and you might feel like you are barely functioning. Brain fog—that feeling of slow thinking, difficulty concentrating, and memory lapses—also often gets worse.

This is not just being tired. It is a physiological consequence of the hormonal changes, the hemodynamic stress, and the immense energy your body is using to build the placenta and the baby.

Radical Acceptance and Rest

The most important strategy for managing this fatigue is radical acceptance. You must rest. This is not laziness. This is a medical necessity.

Stop fighting the fatigue. Stop telling yourself you "should" be able to do more. Stop feeling guilty about resting. Your body is doing incredibly hard work. Listen to it.

Practical Strategies:

- **Pacing:** Break down tasks into small, manageable steps. Take frequent breaks. Use the energy conservation strategies discussed in Chapter 3 (shower chair, stools).

- **Prioritization:** Focus on essential tasks only. Let the non-essential things go. The laundry can wait. The emails can wait.

- **Communicate Needs:** Be clear with your partner, family, and employer about your limitations. This is where the preparation in Chapter 3 pays off.

- **Work Accommodations:** If you are working, you may need accommodations. This might include flexible hours, the ability to work from home, or a temporary reduction in duties. Discuss this with your employer early. Under the Pregnant Workers Fairness Act (PWFA) in the US, employers are required to provide reasonable accommodations.

- **Nutrition:** While difficult with nausea, try to prioritize protein and complex carbohydrates when you can eat, to stabilize energy levels.

The first trimester is about surviving. Give yourself permission to prioritize your health and your pregnancy above all else. The intensity will usually ease as you move into the second trimester.

First Trimester Survival Guide

- **Expect Symptom Flares:** The early hemodynamic changes (vasodilation before blood volume increase) often worsen POTS symptoms. This is normal and usually temporary.

- **Differentiate Nausea:** Understand the difference between morning sickness and POTS-related nausea. Manage nausea aggressively with small meals, B6/ginger, and medications if needed.

- **Be Alert for HG:** POTS patients are at higher risk for Hyperemesis Gravidarum. Seek early intervention for severe nausea and vomiting. Do not wait until you are severely dehydrated.

- **Aggressive Hydration:** Maximize oral fluid and electrolyte intake (small sips, ice chips, high-sodium electrolytes). Establish a plan for IV hydration if oral intake is insufficient.

- **Prioritize Rest:** Accept the extreme fatigue and prioritize rest radically. Communicate your needs, adjust your expectations, and implement work accommodations if necessary.

Chapter 5: The Second Trimester (Weeks 13-27): Blood Volume and Adaptation

The second trimester often brings a welcome shift. For many women with POTS, this is the "golden period." The intense nausea and fatigue of the first trimester often subside, and the physical burden of the late third trimester hasn't started yet.

This chapter focuses on capitalizing on this period of relative stability, adapting your management strategies to the changing mechanics of your body, and addressing the new challenges that emerge as the baby grows. But remember, even if you feel better, you still have POTS. You cannot afford to get complacent.

The impact of increased blood volume (Why some feel better, why others don't)

By the middle of the second trimester, your blood volume is increasing significantly. It's heading towards that 30-50% increase we talked about (Sanghavi & Rutherford, 2014). This is the main physiological reason why many POTS patients feel significantly better during this time.

The Physiology of Improvement:

The extra fluid acts as a natural treatment for POTS, especially if you have hypovolemic POTS (low blood volume). It fills up the blood vessels, improving venous return to the heart. This means the heart doesn't have to work as hard when you stand up. The result? Reduced tachycardia, less dizziness, improved energy levels, and clearer thinking.

Some women feel so good that they might even be able to reduce or temporarily stop their POTS medications (always under medical supervision, of course).

Why Some Don't Feel Better:

However, this improvement is not universal. Some women continue to struggle with severe symptoms throughout the second trimester. If this is you, it can be incredibly discouraging, especially when you hear others talking about how great they feel.

Why does this happen?

- **Severe Vasodilation:** If the relaxation of your blood vessels (vasodilation) caused by pregnancy hormones is very pronounced, the increased blood volume might not be enough to overcome the excessive blood pooling.

- **Hyperadrenergic POTS:** If your POTS is driven by an overactive sympathetic nervous system (high adrenaline/fight-or-flight response), the increased blood volume might not address the underlying issue. You might still experience tachycardia, anxiety, palpitations, and blood pressure spikes.

- **Comorbidities:** If you have other conditions like MCAS or EDS, they might continue to cause symptoms even if your hemodynamics improve. MCAS flares can still occur, and EDS-related pain might increase.

- **Persistent Nausea/HG:** If you are still struggling with nausea or HG, the resulting dehydration will continue to exacerbate POTS symptoms.

It is important to validate both experiences. If you feel better, enjoy it, but stay vigilant with your management strategies. If you don't feel better, it doesn't mean you are doing something wrong. It just means your body needs more support. Continue working closely with your medical team to adjust your treatment plan.

Managing orthostatic intolerance and venous pooling

Even if your overall symptoms improve, *orthostatic intolerance—* the inability to tolerate being upright—remains a core challenge. As the baby grows, new factors come into play that can worsen blood pooling.

The Growing Uterus:

The uterus expands, putting pressure on the veins in your pelvis. This can impede blood flow back to the heart, making *venous pooling* (blood collecting in the lower body) worse, especially when standing still for long periods.

Management Strategies:

You need to double down on your strategies to support circulation.

- **Avoid Prolonged Standing:** This remains the golden rule of POTS management. Use a stool when cooking or showering. Sit down whenever possible. If you have to stand in line, ask for a chair or sit on the floor. Don't worry about what people think.

- **Counter-Maneuvers:** When you do have to stand, use physical counter-maneuvers to activate the muscle pump in your legs and push blood upward.

  - Tense your leg and buttock muscles.

  - Cross your legs while standing.

  - Shift your weight frequently or march in place.

- **Hydration and Salt:** Continue your aggressive hydration and salt intake. Your needs might actually increase as your blood volume expands. Don't slack off just because you feel better.

- **Heat Avoidance:** Heat causes vasodilation and worsens blood pooling. Be extremely careful in hot weather, hot showers, and overheated rooms. Use fans, cooling towels, and stay in air conditioning when possible.

Compression strategies: The necessity of waist-high maternity compression

Compression garments are essential for POTS management. They provide external pressure to the legs, preventing blood pooling and improving circulation. They are arguably one of the most effective non-pharmacological treatments.

During pregnancy, standard knee-high or thigh-high compression often isn't enough. The blood pooling often extends to the abdomen and pelvic area, and the pressure from the growing uterus exacerbates this.

The Importance of Waist-High Compression:

We strongly recommend **waist-high maternity compression stockings** starting in the second trimester (or earlier if needed). These provide support for the entire lower body and the abdomen. Studies show that compression covering the abdomen is more effective at managing orthostatic intolerance than leg compression alone (Bourne et al., 2021).

- **Grade of Compression:** Medical-grade compression (usually 20-30 mmHg or higher) is most effective. The cheap "support hose" or maternity leggings sold in stores do not provide enough pressure to be therapeutically useful for POTS.

- **Fit:** Getting the right fit is crucial and challenging as your body changes. You may need to be professionally measured at a medical supply store. They need to be tight but not painful.

Tips for Tolerating Compression:

Let's be honest: Compression stockings are hot, uncomfortable, and difficult to put on, especially when pregnant. But the benefits usually outweigh the discomfort.

- **Application:** Put them on *before* you get out of bed in the morning. If you wait until you have been standing, the blood has already pooled in your legs, and the stockings will trap it there.

- **Tools:** Use rubber gloves to get a better grip. Use specialized tools (donning aids) to help you pull them on, especially as your belly grows.

- **Material:** Look for breathable materials. Open-toe options might be cooler.

- **Abdominal Binders/Maternity Belts:** Some women find that an abdominal binder or a firm maternity support belt provides additional support and improves circulation, either alone or in combination with compression stockings.

Compression can make a significant difference in managing dizziness, fatigue, leg swelling, and varicose veins. It is a non-negotiable part of your daily uniform.

Exercise modifications: Safe movement (recumbent, swimming) and avoiding supine positions

Physical activity remains crucial in the second trimester. If you are feeling better, this is the time to capitalize on it and maintain or improve your conditioning. Exercise helps manage weight gain, improves mood, and prepares your body for the demands of labor and postpartum recovery. However, your exercise routine needs to be modified as your body changes.

POTS-Friendly Exercises:

Continue focusing on exercises that minimize orthostatic stress, following the principles of the Levine/CHOP protocols (see Chapter 1).

- **Swimming and Water Aerobics:** These are the gold standard for POTS exercise during pregnancy. The hydrostatic pressure of the water acts as natural compression, supporting circulation and reducing tachycardia. The buoyancy also takes the strain off your joints.

- **Recumbent Bike and Rowing Machine:** Still excellent choices for cardiovascular conditioning.

- **Prenatal Yoga and Pilates:** Can help with flexibility and core strength, but be careful with rapid posture changes (e.g., going from bending over to standing up quickly). Modify poses as needed and listen to your body.

Adapting to Pregnancy Changes:

- **Center of Gravity:** Your center of gravity is shifting as your belly grows, which can affect your balance. Be cautious with activities that require significant balance.

- **Joint Laxity:** Pregnancy hormones (relaxin) loosen your joints. If you have EDS or hypermobility, you need to be extra careful to avoid injury and dislocations. Focus on controlled movements and avoid overstretching.

-

Avoiding Supine Positions (Lying Flat on Your Back)

This is critical. After the middle of the second trimester (around 20 weeks), you should avoid lying flat on your back for prolonged periods, including during exercise and sleep.

The weight of the uterus can compress the *vena cava* (the large vein that returns blood from your lower body to your heart). This is known as *supine hypotension syndrome*. It can cause a sudden drop in blood pressure, severe dizziness, shortness of breath, and, importantly, reduced blood flow to the baby.

- **Exercise Modifications:** Modify exercises that are typically done lying flat (like crunches or certain yoga poses) to be done on an incline, seated, or side-lying.

- **Sleeping Position:** Sleep on your side, preferably the left side, which maximizes blood flow. Use pregnancy pillows or wedges for support and comfort.

Work and lifestyle accommodations

By the second trimester, your pregnancy is visible, and you might be feeling the cumulative effects of the physical demands, even if your POTS symptoms are better controlled. This is the time to implement accommodations at work and in your daily life to ensure you can sustain your activity levels without crashing.

Work Accommodations:

If you are working, you may need formal accommodations. As mentioned earlier, employers in the US are required to provide reasonable accommodations for pregnancy (PWFA) and disability (ADA).

Examples of accommodations for POTS during pregnancy:

- **Flexible Hours:** Adjusting your start and end times to avoid peak commute times or manage morning symptoms.

- **Telework:** Working from home to reduce fatigue, manage symptoms, and control your environment.

- **Workspace Modifications:** A desk that allows you to sit or stand, a fan to control temperature, or a location near the restroom.

- **Breaks:** Frequent breaks to rest, hydrate, eat, and change positions.

- **Reduced Standing:** Modifications to job duties to minimize prolonged standing.

Requesting Accommodations:

- **Be Proactive:** Discuss your needs with your employer and HR department early. Don't wait until you are struggling.

- **Provide Documentation:** Get a letter from your MFM or POTS specialist outlining your condition and the specific accommodations needed.

- **Focus on Solutions:** Frame your request in terms of how the accommodations will help you remain productive and healthy.

Lifestyle Adjustments:

Be realistic about your energy levels. The "boom-bust" cycle is still a threat.

- **Social Commitments:** Reduce non-essential social commitments. Learn to say no without guilt. Your priority is your health and the baby.

- **Travel:** Travel can be challenging due to prolonged sitting, dehydration, and changes in routine. If you must travel, plan ahead. Wear compression, hydrate aggressively, and request aisle seats so you can get up and move frequently.

- **Support System:** Activate your support system for help with household tasks and errands. Continue the role definitions discussed in Chapter 3.

Creating a sustainable lifestyle that supports your health and your pregnancy is essential. Stop trying to do everything. Prioritize what matters.

Second Trimester Strategies

- **Understand Blood Volume Changes:** The increase in blood volume often improves POTS symptoms, but this is not universal. Do not get discouraged if you still struggle.

- **Combat Venous Pooling:** Use waist-high medical-grade maternity compression garments daily. Avoid prolonged standing and use counter-maneuvers.

- **Maintain Hydration and Salt:** Do not reduce your fluid and salt intake even if you feel better.

- **Modify Exercise:** Focus on POTS-friendly exercises like swimming and recumbent biking. Avoid exercises that require lying flat on your back (supine position).

- **Implement Accommodations:** Request necessary accommodations at work and adjust your lifestyle to conserve energy and avoid the boom-bust cycle.

Chapter 6: The Third Trimester (Weeks 28-40+): Preparation and Endurance

The third trimester is the home stretch, but it often feels like the longest stretch. The physical demands are intense. The baby is bigger, the strain on your cardiovascular system is greater, and anxiety about delivery often increases. This chapter is about managing these late-pregnancy challenges and preparing logistically and emotionally for the birth.

It's about endurance. You've made it this far. Now you need the strategies to cross the finish line safely and rationally.

Managing increased cardiac demands, tachycardia, and shortness of breath

Your cardiovascular system is working harder than it ever has. It's pumping that extra 50% blood volume to support both you and the baby. It is normal for your resting heart rate to be significantly higher now than it was before pregnancy (often 10-20 bpm higher).

However, for someone with POTS, this increased cardiac demand can lead to more frequent episodes of *tachycardia* (rapid heart rate) and palpitations (feeling like your heart is pounding or fluttering). You might find that activities that were manageable in the second trimester—like walking up a flight of stairs or taking a shower—now cause your heart rate to spike excessively.

Shortness of Breath:

Shortness of breath is also very common in the third trimester. It can be quite uncomfortable and even scary. There are several reasons for this:

1. **Diaphragm Compression:** The growing uterus pushes up on your diaphragm (the muscle below your lungs), reducing the space for your lungs to expand fully.

2. **Increased Cardiac Workload:** The heart is working harder, increasing the demand for oxygen.

3. **POTS-Related "Air Hunger":** POTS patients often experience a feeling of "air hunger" (a sensation of not being able to get a deep breath) even when their oxygen levels are normal. This is related to autonomic dysfunction and changes in respiratory control.

Management Strategies:

- **Pacing:** Slow down. Seriously. Move at a pace that feels comfortable, even if it's very slow. Take breaks frequently. Avoid rushing.

- **Positioning:** Sit upright and supported (e.g., with pillows behind your back) to maximize lung capacity. Sleeping in a semi-reclined position might be more comfortable than lying flat on your side.

- **Cooling:** Heat exacerbates tachycardia and shortness of breath. Use fans, stay in cool environments, and wear light clothing.

- **Medication Adjustments:** If the tachycardia is severe, persistent, and interfering with your function, talk to your medical team. They may recommend adjusting your medication (e.g., increasing the dose of a beta-blocker) if it is safe to do so.

When to Worry:

While these symptoms are common, they can sometimes indicate a more serious problem, such as severe anemia (which reduces oxygen-carrying capacity) or a cardiac issue (like pulmonary embolism or peripartum cardiomyopathy, although these are rare).

It is crucial to report any significant changes in your symptoms to your MFM. If you experience sudden onset of severe shortness of breath, chest pain, rapid, irregular heartbeat, or coughing up blood, seek medical attention immediately. Don't dismiss it as "just POTS."

Positioning challenges and managing supine hypotension syndrome

As discussed in Chapter 5, lying flat on your back is a major problem in late pregnancy. *Supine hypotension syndrome*—where the heavy uterus compresses the vena cava, reducing blood flow back to the heart—becomes much more pronounced and common in the third trimester.

This is not just uncomfortable; it is dangerous. It can cause a sudden drop in blood pressure, severe dizziness, nausea, and, critically, reduced blood flow to the placenta and the baby.

Safe Positioning Strategies:

- **Side-Lying:** Sleeping and resting on your side (preferably the left side, which optimizes blood flow) is the safest position. Use multiple pillows or a large pregnancy pillow to support your back, belly, hips, and knees.

- **Incline/Wedge:** If you must be on your back for a short period (e.g., during an ultrasound or non-stress test), ensure you are on an incline (at least 30 degrees) or have a wedge placed under your right hip to tilt the uterus off the vena cava. This is called *left uterine displacement.*

- **Semi-Reclined:** Resting in a recliner chair is often comfortable and safe, as long as you are not completely flat.

Communicating Your Needs:

Be vocal and assertive about your positioning needs during medical appointments. If a technician asks you to lie flat, remind them that you cannot due to the risk of supine hypotension. Ask for a wedge or to be positioned on your side.

If you start to feel dizzy, short of breath, or nauseous while lying down, tell the provider immediately and shift to your side. Do not try to tolerate it.

Fall prevention and managing pre-syncope

Pre-syncope (the feeling that you are about to faint) can become more frequent in the third trimester. There are several reasons for this: your center of gravity is off, you are likely exhausted, orthostatic stress is high, and the physical burden of the pregnancy can exacerbate blood pooling.

Fainting (syncope) while pregnant is dangerous. A fall can injure you and the baby, and potentially lead to serious complications like placental abruption (where the placenta detaches from the uterine wall).

Fall Prevention is Critical:

You must take precautions to prevent falls.

- **Move Slowly:** Get up slowly from a lying or sitting position. Sit on the edge of the bed for a few minutes before standing. Do not rush.

- **Use Support:** Always have something nearby to hold onto when standing. Use handrails on stairs (have someone walk behind you if possible).

- **Mobility Aids:** If you are feeling very unstable, use a cane, walker, or rollator (a walker with a seat). There is absolutely no shame in this. Safety is the priority. Swallow your pride and use the tools you need.

- **Shower Safety:** Continue using a shower chair and avoid hot showers. Have someone nearby when you are showering if possible.

- **Home Environment:** Remove tripping hazards (like throw rugs, clutter, or cords) from your home. Use nightlights.

- **Listen to Your Body:** If you feel dizzy, sit down immediately, wherever you are. Do not try to push through it.

If you do faint, you must contact your MFM immediately, even if you do not think you are injured. They will need to monitor the baby (usually with a non-stress test) to ensure everything is okay.

Detailed birth planning: Creating the POTS Birth Plan

You need a birth plan. But not the typical birth plan that focuses on music, lighting, and aromatherapy. You need a **POTS-Specific Birth Plan**.

This document communicates your essential medical needs to the labor and delivery team (nurses, residents, attending physicians). Remember, the team caring for you in the hospital might not be familiar with POTS. They are busy and often rotating shifts. You need to educate them quickly and clearly.

Your birth plan should be concise (ideally one page), easy to read (use bullet points), and focused on safety essentials related to your autonomic function.

Key Elements of a POTS Birth Plan:

1. **Diagnosis and Brief Description:** Clearly state your diagnosis and how it affects you. (e.g., "I have POTS, an autonomic

disorder that causes severe tachycardia and blood pressure instability when upright. I am at high risk for hypotension.")

2. **Hydration Requirements:** Specify the need for **immediate IV fluids** (e.g., Normal Saline or Lactated Ringers) upon admission to the hospital, even before labor is active. Maintaining blood volume is critical to prevent hemodynamic instability during labor.

3. **Anesthesia Considerations:** Reference your anesthesia consultation. Include the plan for pre-loading with fluids before the epidural and managing hypotension (e.g., preferred vasopressors).

4. **Positioning:** Emphasize the need to avoid lying flat on your back (supine hypotension). Specify the need for left uterine displacement during monitoring and procedures. List preferred positions for labor and delivery (e.g., side-lying, hands and knees).

5. **Monitoring:** Acknowledge the need for continuous cardiac (heart rate and blood pressure) and fetal monitoring.

6. **Medications:** List your current medications and the plan for taking them during labor (e.g., continuing beta-blockers).

7. **Triggers:** List your main triggers (e.g., heat, prolonged standing) and strategies to avoid them (e.g., keeping the room cool, minimizing vaginal exams).

Discussing the Birth Plan:

Review the birth plan with your MFM well before your due date (around 34-36 weeks). Make sure they agree with the plan and that it is documented in your hospital chart. Bring multiple copies of the plan with you to the hospital and give one to your labor nurse at each shift change.

(A detailed template is provided in Part V: The Toolkit).

Hospital preparations: The POTS-specific "Go-Bag" and provider communication

Packing your hospital bag needs a POTS twist. In addition to the usual items (comfortable clothes, toiletries, baby clothes), you need your POTS management essentials. The hospital might not have what you need, or it might take time to get it.

The POTS-Specific "Go-Bag":

- **Electrolytes:** Bring your preferred electrolyte powders or tablets. Hospital options are often limited (e.g., they might only have sugary sports drinks).

- **Salty Snacks:** Easy-to-eat salty snacks (pretzels, nuts) to maintain sodium levels during labor (if allowed) and postpartum.

- **Compression Garments:** Bring your compression stockings or abdominal binder for use immediately after delivery (this is crucial for managing the postpartum hemodynamic shift).

- **Water Bottle:** A large water bottle with a straw, so you can drink easily while lying down.

- **Portable Fan:** Hospitals can be warm, and heat intolerance is common during labor and postpartum. A small battery-operated or USB fan can be a lifesaver.

- **Medical Information:** Copies of your birth plan, medical summary, and emergency contact list.

Final Provider Communication:

In the weeks leading up to your due date, ensure all your providers are on the same page.

- Confirm that your MFM has communicated the birth plan and any specific orders to the hospital labor and delivery unit.

- Discuss the plan for induction if necessary. Some induction methods (like certain cervical ripening agents) can affect hemodynamics or trigger mast cell reactions if you have MCAS.

- Review the emergency procedures and ensure your partner is prepared to advocate for you during labor if you are unable to communicate effectively.

Preparation is the antidote to anxiety. By anticipating the challenges and having a clear plan in place, you can approach your birth with confidence and focus on the task at hand: bringing your baby safely into the world.

Third Trimester Checklist

- **Manage Cardiac Demands:** Use pacing, positioning, and cooling strategies to manage tachycardia and shortness of breath. Report any sudden or severe changes to your MFM.

- **Avoid Supine Positions:** Strictly avoid lying flat on your back. Sleep on your side or semi-reclined. Ensure left uterine displacement during monitoring and procedures.

- **Prioritize Fall Prevention:** Move slowly, use support, and utilize mobility aids if needed. Sit down immediately if you feel dizzy.

- **Create a POTS-Specific Birth Plan:** Focus on IV hydration, anesthesia considerations, and positioning. Review it with your MFM and bring copies to the hospital.

- **Prepare Your Hospital Bag:** Pack your POTS essentials, including electrolytes, compression gear, a fan, and medical information.

Chapter 7: Labor and Delivery Strategies

Labor and delivery are intense physical events. They place significant stress on the cardiovascular and autonomic nervous systems. For someone with POTS, this is the ultimate stress test. But you are not going into it unprepared. You have a plan.

This chapter focuses on the specific strategies for managing POTS during labor and delivery. The goal is to maintain hemodynamic stability (stable heart rate and blood pressure) to ensure the safety of both you and the baby.

Physiological challenges of labor with dysautonomia

Labor is dynamic. It involves pain, stress, fluid shifts, and intense physical exertion. All of these factors directly impact autonomic function.

Pain and Stress:

Pain and anxiety activate the sympathetic nervous system (fight-or-flight response). This can trigger adrenaline surges, leading to increased tachycardia, palpitations, and potentially blood pressure spikes (especially if you have hyperadrenergic POTS). Managing pain effectively is not just about comfort; it is about maintaining autonomic stability.

Fluid Shifts:

You might lose fluids through sweating, vomiting, or bleeding during labor. Dehydration can quickly worsen POTS symptoms and lead to hypotension (low blood pressure). Maintaining adequate hydration is critical.

Positional Changes:

You might be asked to change positions frequently during labor. Moving from lying down to sitting or standing can trigger orthostatic stress. Certain positions (like lying flat on your back) can cause supine hypotension syndrome (see Chapter 6).

Physical Exertion (Pushing):

The pushing stage of labor involves intense physical exertion and the Valsalva maneuver (bearing down). This maneuver causes rapid changes in blood pressure and heart rate. For some POTS patients, this can trigger severe dizziness, pre-syncope, or even fainting.

Medications:

Medications used during labor (such asPitocin for induction or certain pain medications) can also affect hemodynamics.

Understanding these challenges allows you to anticipate them and implement strategies to mitigate their impact.

Fluid management: The critical role of IV hydration protocols during labor

Aggressive fluid management is arguably the most important intervention for managing POTS during labor and delivery. It is essential for maintaining blood volume, preventing dehydration, and stabilizing blood pressure.

The Need for IV Fluids:

Oral hydration is usually not sufficient during labor due to the intensity of the physical demands and the potential for nausea and vomiting. You need intravenous (IV) fluids.

IV Hydration Protocol:

- **Early Administration:** IV fluids should be started as soon as you are admitted to the hospital, even if you are not yet in active labor. Do not wait until you are dehydrated.

- **Type of Fluid:** Normal Saline (0.9% sodium chloride) or Lactated Ringer's solution are typically used. These isotonic solutions help expand blood volume effectively.

- **Rate of Administration:** The rate of IV fluids will be determined by your medical team based on your hydration status, vital signs, and the stage of labor. A continuous infusion is usually necessary.

- **Fluid Boluses:** Additional rapid infusions of fluid (boluses) might be needed before anesthesia administration (see below) or if your blood pressure drops.

Advocacy:

Make sure your need for early and continuous IV hydration is clearly stated in your birth plan. Your partner should also be prepared to advocate for this if there is any delay.

Case Example: Keeping an Eye on the Fluids

Emily arrived at the hospital in early labor. Her nurse was busy and didn't start her IV fluids right away, despite it being in her birth plan. Emily started feeling dizzy and her heart rate increased. Her husband reminded the nurse about the IV fluids. The nurse started the infusion, and within an hour, Emily's symptoms improved significantly. Maintaining that hydration throughout her labor helped her manage the physical stress effectively.

Anesthesia considerations: Epidurals, spinal blocks, and managing hemodynamic instability risks

Pain management is a major concern for women with POTS during labor. As mentioned earlier, pain can trigger adrenaline surges and worsen autonomic instability. An epidural is often the most effective method of pain relief. However, it also poses specific risks for POTS patients.

The Risk of Hypotension:

Epidurals and spinal blocks work by blocking the nerve signals in the lower body. This includes the sympathetic nerves that control vasoconstriction (tightening of blood vessels). As a result, these procedures cause vasodilation (widening of blood vessels) in the lower body.

This leads to a sudden drop in blood pressure (*hypotension*). In POTS patients, who already have difficulty regulating blood pressure, this drop can be dramatic and rapid. Severe hypotension can cause fainting and reduce blood flow to the baby.

Strategies for Safe Anesthesia:

Epidurals are not contraindicated in POTS, but they must be managed carefully by an experienced anesthesiologist who understands your condition. This is why the pre-delivery anesthesia consultation (Chapter 2) is so important.

The plan for safe anesthesia should include:

- **IV Fluid Pre-loading:** You must receive a significant amount of IV fluids (usually 1-2 liters) rapidly *before* the epidural is placed. This expands your blood volume to counteract the vasodilation.

- **Slow Dosing:** The anesthesiologist should administer the medication slowly and in small doses to minimize the hemodynamic impact.

- **Close Monitoring:** Your blood pressure and heart rate must be monitored closely (often every 1-2 minutes) immediately after the epidural is placed.

- **Vasopressors:** Medications that raise blood pressure (vasopressors), such as phenylephrine or ephedrine, must be readily available and administered promptly if hypotension occurs.

- **Positioning:** You must maintain left uterine displacement (tilted to the side) after the epidural is placed to prevent supine hypotension syndrome.

Other Pain Management Options:

If an epidural is not possible or desired, other options include:

- **Nitrous Oxide ("Laughing Gas"):** Can help reduce anxiety and pain without significant hemodynamic effects.

- **IV Pain Medications:** Opioids can be used, but they can sometimes cause nausea or sedation.

- **Non-Pharmacological Methods:** Breathing techniques, massage, hydrotherapy (if available and safe), and movement can also be helpful.

The key is to have a plan and to communicate effectively with your anesthesia team.

Positioning options to minimize orthostatic stress

Your position during labor and delivery can significantly impact your symptoms and the progress of labor. You need to find positions that minimize orthostatic stress and maximize comfort and safety.

Avoiding Supine Position:

As emphasized repeatedly, avoid lying flat on your back. This position causes supine hypotension syndrome and should be avoided at all costs.

Optimal Labor Positions:

- **Side-Lying:** Often the most comfortable and hemodynamically stable position. It allows you to rest while minimizing pressure on the vena cava.

- **Hands and Knees:** Can help relieve back pain and improve fetal positioning.

- **Seated/Semi-Reclined:** If you are sitting up, ensure you are well-supported and not completely upright, which can increase orthostatic stress.

Positioning During Pushing:

The traditional position of lying on your back with your legs in stirrups is often the worst position for POTS patients. Discuss alternative pushing positions with your MFM.

- **Side-Lying Pushing:** Very effective and minimizes hemodynamic stress.

- **Supported Squatting or Sitting:** Can be effective but might be too physically demanding if you are fatigued.

Mobility During Labor:

If you are able to walk (and do not have an epidural), frequent movement can help progress labor. However, you must be careful to avoid falls. Have someone assist you when you are upright.

If you have an epidural, you will be confined to the bed, but you should still change positions frequently (e.g., alternating sides) with the help of your nurse and partner.

Monitoring requirements (Cardiac and Fetal)

Because POTS is considered a high-risk condition, you will require continuous monitoring during labor and delivery.

Fetal Monitoring:

Continuous electronic fetal monitoring (EFM) is standard to ensure the baby is tolerating labor well. This involves wearing belts around your abdomen to monitor the baby's heart rate and your contractions.

Maternal Monitoring:

- **Vital Signs:** Your heart rate, blood pressure, and oxygen saturation will be monitored frequently.

- **ECG (Electrocardiogram):** In some cases, your medical team may recommend continuous ECG monitoring (telemetry) to monitor your heart rhythm, especially if you have a history of significant arrhythmias.

Managing Monitoring Challenges:

Continuous monitoring can be restrictive and uncomfortable. The belts can be tight, and the constant noise of the machines can be stressful.

- **Positioning:** Ensure the monitors are placed correctly so they do not interfere with your preferred positions.

- **Wireless Monitoring:** Some hospitals offer wireless monitoring systems that allow for more freedom of movement. Ask if this is available.

- **Communication:** If you are feeling overwhelmed by the monitoring, communicate your concerns to your nurse.

Monitoring is essential for safety. It allows the medical team to detect any signs of distress early and intervene promptly.

Labor and Delivery Playbook

- **Understand the Challenges:** Pain, stress, fluid shifts, and physical exertion during labor can exacerbate autonomic instability.

- **Prioritize IV Hydration:** Start IV fluids immediately upon admission and maintain continuous infusion throughout labor.

- **Manage Anesthesia Risks:** Epidurals can cause severe hypotension. Ensure IV fluid pre-loading, slow dosing, close monitoring, and availability of vasopressors.

- **Optimize Positioning:** Avoid lying flat on your back. Use side-lying and other positions that minimize orthostatic stress during labor and pushing.

- **Expect Continuous Monitoring:** Continuous fetal and maternal monitoring (heart rate, blood pressure) is necessary for safety.

Chapter 8: Cesarean Birth and Surgical Considerations

While the goal is often a vaginal delivery, sometimes a Cesarean birth (C-section) is necessary for the safety of the mother or the baby. About one-third of births in the US are C-sections. It is important to understand the specific considerations for C-sections when you have POTS, as surgery poses unique challenges for autonomic function.

This chapter covers the POTS-specific risks associated with C-sections, the anesthesia management strategies, and the modifications needed for a safe recovery.

Indications and POTS-specific surgical risks

A C-section might be planned (scheduled in advance) or unplanned (emergent during labor).

Common Indications for C-section:

- Fetal distress (the baby is not tolerating labor well).

- Breech presentation (the baby is positioned feet or buttocks first).

- Placenta previa (the placenta is covering the cervix).

- Failure to progress (labor is stalled).

POTS-Specific Considerations:

In some cases, a C-section might be recommended if the mother's POTS symptoms are so severe that she cannot tolerate the physical exertion of labor and pushing. However, this is relatively rare. Most women with POTS can safely deliver vaginally with appropriate management.

Surgical Risks Associated with POTS:

Surgery, including C-sections, involves several factors that can destabilize autonomic function:

- **Anesthesia:** As discussed in Chapter 7, anesthesia (spinal or epidural) can cause significant hypotension. General anesthesia (being put to sleep) also carries risks and is usually avoided unless absolutely necessary.

- **Fluid Shifts and Blood Loss:** C-sections typically involve more blood loss than vaginal deliveries. Even a normal amount of blood loss can be poorly tolerated by POTS patients, who may already have low blood volume or be sensitive to fluid shifts.

- **Positioning:** During surgery, you are typically lying flat on your back. Although the operating table is tilted to the side (left uterine displacement) to prevent supine hypotension syndrome, this position can still be challenging.

- **Post-Surgical Immobility:** Being immobile after surgery increases the risk of deconditioning and blood clots.

Comorbidities and Surgical Risks:

If you have comorbidities like EDS or MCAS, the surgical risks are further complicated.

- **EDS:** Increased risk of wound healing problems, excessive bleeding, and potential resistance to local anesthetics.

- **MCAS:** Risk of allergic reactions or mast cell degranulation triggered by medications, surgical materials, or the stress of surgery.

It is crucial that your surgical team (MFM, anesthesiologist) is aware of all your diagnoses and has a plan to manage these risks.

Anesthesia management during a C-section

The principles of anesthesia management during a C-section are similar to those discussed in Chapter 7, but the implementation is often more urgent, especially in an unplanned C-section.

Spinal Anesthesia (Spinal Block):

This is the most common type of anesthesia used for planned C-sections. It involves injecting medication into the spinal fluid, causing rapid numbness from the chest down.

- **Risks:** Spinal blocks often cause a faster and more profound drop in blood pressure than epidurals.

- **Management:** Aggressive IV fluid pre-loading (1-2 liters) is essential. Vasopressors (like phenylephrine) are often administered prophylactically (before the blood pressure drops) or immediately if hypotension occurs.

Epidural Anesthesia:

If you already have a working epidural during labor and need an unplanned C-section, the anesthesiologist can usually increase the dose of medication through the epidural catheter to achieve surgical anesthesia.

- **Benefits:** The onset of hypotension is usually slower than with a spinal block, allowing more time for intervention.

General Anesthesia:

General anesthesia is usually reserved for emergencies when there is no time for a spinal or epidural, or if regional anesthesia is contraindicated.

- **Risks:** Can cause significant hemodynamic instability during induction (going to sleep) and emergence (waking up). Also poses risks for the baby (respiratory depression).

Communication is Key:

If you are having a C-section, communicate your concerns and needs to the anesthesia team. Remind them about your POTS diagnosis and your sensitivity to hypotension. Ask them about their plan for managing your blood pressure.

If you start feeling dizzy, nauseous, or short of breath during the surgery, tell the anesthesiologist immediately. These are often signs of dropping blood pressure.

Post-surgical recovery modifications: Pain management, mobility, and compression

Recovery from a C-section is more challenging than recovery from a vaginal delivery. It is major abdominal surgery. For POTS patients, the recovery process requires specific modifications to manage symptoms and prevent complications.

Pain Management:

Effective pain management is crucial. Pain activates the sympathetic nervous system and worsens POTS symptoms. It also interferes with mobility and rest.

- **Multimodal Analgesia:** A combination of medications is usually used, including opioids, NSAIDs (like ibuprofen), and acetaminophen.

- **POTS Considerations:** Some pain medications can cause nausea, constipation, or sedation, which can exacerbate POTS symptoms. Communicate with your team about how you are tolerating the medications.

- **Non-Pharmacological Methods:** Use ice packs on the incision site and supportive pillows for comfort.

Mobility Planning:

Early mobilization (getting up and moving) is essential after a C-section to prevent blood clots, promote healing, and prevent deconditioning. However, this can be extremely difficult for POTS patients due to pain and orthostatic intolerance.

- **Gradual Progression:** Start slowly. Begin by sitting up in bed, then dangling your legs over the side, then standing with assistance.

- **Assistance:** You will need help getting out of bed for the first few days. Do not try to do it alone.

- **Orthostatic Precautions:** When you stand up, do it slowly. Be alert for signs of dizziness or pre-syncope.

- **Short, Frequent Walks:** Aim for short, frequent walks around the room or the hospital unit, rather than long periods of activity.

Compression Protocols:

Compression is critical after a C-section to manage orthostatic intolerance and prevent blood clots.

- **SCDs (Sequential Compression Devices):** These are inflatable sleeves placed on your legs while you are in bed to promote circulation and prevent blood clots. Use them consistently.

- **Abdominal Binder:** Many women find that an abdominal binder provides support for the incision site and also helps manage orthostatic intolerance by reducing abdominal blood pooling. Ask your nurse for one.

- **Compression Stockings:** You should resume wearing your compression stockings as soon as possible after surgery.

Preventing deconditioning post-surgery

Deconditioning (loss of muscle mass and cardiovascular fitness) happens rapidly with immobility. Even a few days of bed rest can significantly worsen POTS symptoms. Preventing deconditioning is a major goal of post-surgical recovery.

- **Early Mobilization:** As discussed above, getting moving early and often is the most effective strategy.

- **Physical Therapy:** A consultation with a physical therapist in the hospital can be helpful. They can teach you exercises you can do in bed (like ankle pumps and leg lifts) and help you with safe mobilization techniques.

- **Nutrition and Hydration:** Adequate nutrition (especially protein) and hydration are essential for healing and maintaining energy levels. Continue your high salt and fluid intake (adjusting for any IV fluids you are receiving).

- **Rest and Pacing:** While mobilization is important, rest is also crucial for healing. Balance activity with rest. Listen to your body and do not push yourself too hard.

Recovery from a C-section with POTS is a marathon, not a sprint. Be patient with yourself, follow the recommended protocols, and ask for help when you need it.

C-Section Strategies

- **Understand the Risks:** C-sections pose specific risks for POTS patients, including hypotension, blood loss, and post-surgical immobility. Comorbidities like EDS and MCAS further complicate these risks.

- **Optimize Anesthesia Management:** Spinal or epidural anesthesia requires aggressive IV fluid pre-loading and prompt management of hypotension with vasopressors.

- **Modify Recovery:** Focus on effective pain management, gradual mobilization with assistance, and consistent use of compression (SCDs, abdominal binder, stockings).

- **Prevent Deconditioning:** Prioritize early mobilization, physical therapy, adequate nutrition and hydration, and balanced rest and pacing.

Chapter 9: The Fourth Trimester: The Critical First 12 Weeks

You did it. You made it through the pregnancy and delivery. The baby is here. Now the real work begins. The "fourth trimester" (the first 12 weeks postpartum) is often the most challenging period for women with POTS.

While the focus shifts to the newborn, your body is undergoing another massive physiological transformation. The hormonal shifts are dramatic, the physical demands are intense, and the sleep deprivation is brutal. All of these factors can trigger significant POTS flares.

This chapter is about preparing for and managing the realities of the fourth trimester. It's about prioritizing your recovery while caring for your newborn.

The postpartum hemodynamic shift: Managing the blood volume drop and intense orthostatic stress

During pregnancy, your blood volume increased by up to 50%. This extra fluid often helped stabilize your POTS symptoms. Immediately after delivery, this changes rapidly.

The Blood Volume Drop:

- **Blood Loss:** You lose blood during delivery (even a normal amount can be significant for POTS patients).

- **Diuresis:** Your body starts to shed the excess fluid accumulated during pregnancy through frequent urination and sweating.

This rapid drop in blood volume means your POTS symptoms—especially orthostatic intolerance (dizziness, tachycardia upon standing)—often return with a vengeance in the days and weeks after delivery. You might feel worse than you did before pregnancy.

Managing the Hemodynamic Shift:

- **Aggressive Hydration and Salt:** You need to continue your high salt and fluid intake (2.5-3 liters/day, 7+ grams of salt/day). This is crucial for replenishing your blood volume.

- **Compression:** Wear your waist-high compression stockings and/or an abdominal binder consistently, especially when upright. This is non-negotiable.

- **IV Hydration:** If your symptoms are severe and you are struggling to stay hydrated orally (especially if you are breastfeeding), you may need supplemental IV fluids. Discuss this with your MFM or POTS specialist.

- **Iron Supplementation:** If you lost a significant amount of blood during delivery or are anemic, you may need aggressive iron supplementation (oral or IV infusions) to rebuild your red blood cells and improve energy levels.

Recognizing and managing postpartum flares

A POTS flare postpartum is characterized by a significant worsening of your baseline symptoms. This might include increased dizziness, fainting, extreme fatigue, brain fog, nausea, and tachycardia.

Flares can be triggered by:

- The hemodynamic shift (blood volume drop).

- Sleep deprivation.

- Stress.

- Hormonal fluctuations.

- Infection (e.g., urinary tract infection, mastitis).

Managing Postpartum Flares:

- **Rest:** Prioritize rest whenever possible. This is incredibly difficult with a newborn, but it is essential. (See strategies below).

- **Back to Basics:** Double down on your basic management strategies: hydration, salt, compression.

- **Medication Adjustments:** You may need to adjust your medications (see below).

- **Seek Medical Attention:** If the flare is severe or accompanied by new symptoms (fever, severe pain), contact your doctor immediately to rule out other complications.

Be patient with yourself. It takes time for your body to stabilize after pregnancy and delivery.

Breastfeeding/Chestfeeding with POTS: Hydration needs, positioning, and medication resumption/safety

Breastfeeding or chestfeeding can be a wonderful experience, but it also poses specific challenges for people with POTS.

Hydration Needs:

Breastfeeding increases your fluid needs significantly. You need enough fluid to maintain your own blood volume and produce milk. Dehydration is a major risk.

- **Increase Fluid Intake:** Aim for at least 3-4 liters of fluid per day.

- **Electrolytes:** Continue your high salt intake to retain the fluid.

- **Hydrate While Nursing:** Drink a large glass of fluid every time you nurse. Keep a hydration station next to your nursing chair.

Positioning:

Sitting upright to nurse can trigger orthostatic stress, especially in the early weeks.

- **Side-Lying Nursing:** Nursing while lying on your side is often the most comfortable and hemodynamically stable position.

- **Reclined Nursing:** Nursing in a semi-reclined position with good support can also be effective.

- **Support:** Use pillows to support your arms, back, and the baby, so you are not straining your muscles.

Medication Resumption/Safety:

If you stopped or reduced your POTS medications during pregnancy, you may need to resume them postpartum to manage your symptoms. The safety of medications during breastfeeding is different from pregnancy safety.

- **Beta-Blockers:** Generally considered safe during breastfeeding. Propranolol and Metoprolol are preferred (LactMed, n.d.).

- **Fludrocortisone:** Generally considered safe.

- **Midodrine:** Limited data, but likely safe in small doses.

- **Ivabradine:** Limited data; usually avoided if possible.

Consult with Specialists:

Discuss your medication plan with your POTS specialist and your baby's pediatrician. They can help you weigh the risks and benefits.

Resources like the Drugs and Lactation Database (LactMed) can provide up-to-date information on medication safety.

Formula Feeding is Okay Too:

If breastfeeding is too physically demanding or if you need medications that are not safe during breastfeeding, formula feeding is a perfectly healthy alternative. Your health matters too. A healthy mother is more important than breast milk.

Sleep deprivation strategies and prioritizing maternal rest

Sleep deprivation is inevitable with a newborn. But for POTS patients, lack of sleep is not just tiring; it is a major trigger for symptom flares. It worsens cognitive function, increases stress hormones, and destabilizes autonomic function.

Strategies for Maximizing Sleep:

- **Sleep in Shifts:** If you have a partner, arrange sleep shifts so that each of you gets at least a 4-5 hour stretch of uninterrupted sleep. For example, one person handles feedings from 8pm-1am, and the other handles feedings from 1am-6am.

- **Nap When the Baby Sleeps:** This advice is cliché but crucial. Do not use the baby's nap time to do chores. Rest.

- **Simplify Routines:** Minimize non-essential tasks. Use paper plates. Let the laundry pile up.

- **Limit Visitors:** Visitors can be exhausting. Limit visits to short periods and do not feel obligated to entertain.

Prioritizing Maternal Rest:

You need to prioritize your rest aggressively. This means asking for and accepting help.

- **Partner Support:** Your partner needs to take on a significant share of the newborn care and household responsibilities.

- **Family and Friends:** Ask family and friends for help with meals, errands, or watching the baby while you rest.

- **Hired Help:** If financially feasible, hire help. A postpartum doula, a cleaning service, or a meal delivery service can make a huge difference.

Activating the postpartum support system: Practical and emotional needs

You cannot do this alone. You need a village. This is the time to activate the support system you prepared in Chapter 3.

Practical Support:

Be specific about what you need. People want to help but often don't know how.

- **Meals:** Ask for healthy, easy-to-eat meals. Set up a meal train.

- **Household Tasks:** Ask for help with cleaning, laundry, and grocery shopping.

- **Newborn Care:** Ask someone you trust to watch the baby while you shower, nap, or take a break.

Emotional Support:

The postpartum period is emotionally vulnerable. You are dealing with hormonal shifts, physical recovery, and the stress of new parenthood.

- **Therapy:** Continue seeing your therapist. This is crucial for managing anxiety, processing the birth experience, and adjusting to your new role.

- **Support Groups:** Connect with other new parents, especially those with chronic illnesses. Online groups can be a lifeline.

- **Partner Communication:** Keep the lines of communication open with your partner. Be honest about your feelings and needs.

Monitoring Mental Health:

Be aware of the signs of Perinatal Mood and Anxiety Disorders (PMADs), such as postpartum depression or anxiety. These are common and treatable. If you are struggling with persistent sadness, irritability, intrusive thoughts, or panic attacks, seek help immediately.

The fourth trimester is about survival and adaptation. Be gentle with yourself. Lower your expectations. Focus on the essentials: your recovery and your baby's well-being.

Fourth Trimester Survival

- **Manage the Hemodynamic Shift:** The postpartum drop in blood volume often triggers severe POTS flares. Continue aggressive hydration, salt intake, and compression.

- **Prepare for Flares:** Expect flares triggered by sleep deprivation, stress, and hormonal shifts. Go back to basics and adjust medications as needed.

- **Navigate Breastfeeding Challenges:** Increase fluid and electrolyte intake significantly if breastfeeding. Use side-lying or reclined positions to minimize orthostatic stress.

- **Prioritize Rest:** Implement sleep deprivation strategies (sleep shifts, napping). Aggressively prioritize maternal rest over non-essential tasks.

- **Activate Your Support System:** Ask for and accept practical and emotional support. Monitor your mental health closely and seek help if needed.

Chapter 10: Long-term Recovery and The New Normal

The first year postpartum is a journey of recovery and adjustment. Your body is slowly finding its new equilibrium, and you are learning how to navigate parenthood with a chronic illness. This chapter focuses on the long-term strategies for managing POTS postpartum, building sustainable routines, and embracing your new normal.

Understanding long-term symptom pattern changes

How will your POTS be long-term after pregnancy? This is a common question, and the answer is variable.

Some women find that their POTS symptoms improve long-term after pregnancy. Others return to their pre-pregnancy baseline. And some find that their symptoms are worse, at least for the first year or two.

A recent study found that at 3 months postpartum, nearly 60% of women reported worse symptoms compared to their pre-pregnancy baseline (Dangel et al., 2023). This highlights the intensity of the early postpartum period.

Factors Influencing Long-Term Recovery:

- **Pre-pregnancy Severity:** If your POTS was well-managed before pregnancy, you are more likely to recover well.

- **Pregnancy Complications:** Complications like HG or severe deconditioning during pregnancy can prolong recovery.

- **Postpartum Management:** How aggressively you manage your symptoms and prioritize your recovery in the fourth trimester impacts long-term outcomes.

- **Hormonal Changes:** Fluctuations in hormones (especially if breastfeeding) can continue to affect autonomic function.

It is important to have realistic expectations. Recovery takes time. It is not linear. You will have good days and bad days.

Pacing and energy conservation with newborn

Pacing and energy conservation are essential skills for managing POTS. They become even more critical when you are caring for a newborn who demands constant attention and physical effort.

The Energy Drain of Newborn Care:

Caring for a newborn involves frequent bending, lifting, carrying, and standing. These activities can trigger orthostatic stress and quickly deplete your energy reserves.

Energy Conservation Strategies:

- **Modify Your Environment:** Set up changing stations and feeding stations so that everything you need is within easy reach.

- **Sit Down Whenever Possible:** Sit down while feeding, changing, and playing with the baby.

- **Babywearing:** Using a baby carrier can help distribute the baby's weight and keep your hands free, but be careful with your posture and balance. Ensure the carrier provides adequate support.

- **Break Down Tasks:** Break down tasks into small, manageable steps. Don't try to do everything at once.

- **Prioritize Ruthlessly:** Focus on the essentials (feeding the baby, your own basic needs). Let everything else go.

The "Boom-Bust" Cycle:

Avoid the temptation to overdo it on good days. This leads to the "boom-bust" cycle (overactivity followed by a crash), which hinders long-term recovery. Consistency is key.

Building new routines

Your old routines are gone. You need to build new routines that accommodate the demands of parenthood and the needs of your chronic illness.

- **Flexible Structure:** Create a flexible structure for your day that includes time for rest, hydration, meals, and gentle activity.

- **Hydration Routine:** Integrate hydration into your daily routine. Keep water bottles everywhere.

- **Meal Planning:** Plan simple, healthy meals that require minimal preparation. Use grocery delivery or ask for help with cooking.

- **Support Schedule:** Schedule help from your partner, family, or hired help.

Building new routines takes time and experimentation. Be flexible and adjust as needed.

Gradual physical reconditioning and pelvic floor rehabilitation

Physical reconditioning is crucial for long-term POTS management. Once you are cleared by your doctor (usually around 6 weeks postpartum), you can gradually resume exercise.

Gradual Progression:

Start slowly. You are likely deconditioned from the pregnancy and delivery.

- **Walking:** Begin with short, slow walks.

- **Recumbent Exercise:** Resume recumbent exercises (bike, rowing) at a low intensity and duration.

- **Strength Training:** Focus on rebuilding core and lower body strength.

Physical Therapy:

Working with a physical therapist experienced in POTS can help you develop a safe and effective reconditioning program.

Pelvic Floor Rehabilitation:

Pelvic floor rehabilitation is essential after pregnancy and delivery, especially if you have EDS or experienced tearing. A pelvic floor physical therapist can help you regain strength and function, and address issues like incontinence or pain.

Mental health: Monitoring for Perinatal Mood and Anxiety Disorders (PMADs)

The risk of Perinatal Mood and Anxiety Disorders (PMADs), such as postpartum depression (PPD) and postpartum anxiety (PPA), remains high throughout the first year postpartum. Chronic illness increases this risk.

Recognizing PMADs:

Symptoms of PMADs can overlap with POTS symptoms (fatigue, brain fog), making diagnosis challenging. Look for:

- Persistent sadness, hopelessness, or irritability.

- Loss of interest in activities you usually enjoy.

- Difficulty bonding with the baby.

- Excessive worry or intrusive thoughts.

- Panic attacks.

- Thoughts of self-harm or suicide.

Seeking Help:

If you are struggling, seek help immediately. PMADs are treatable. Contact your doctor or a mental health professional.

Ongoing Support:

Continue therapy and utilize your support network. Taking care of your mental health is essential for your well-being and your ability to care for your baby.

Relationship adjustments and ongoing communication

Having a baby changes your relationship with your partner. Add a chronic illness to the mix, and the challenges are magnified.

- **Communication:** Continue the open and honest communication strategies discussed in Chapter 3. Schedule regular check-ins to discuss how you are both doing.

- **Division of Labor:** Reassess the division of labor regularly. Ensure it is fair and sustainable.

- **Intimacy:** Physical and emotional intimacy might change. Be patient and communicate your needs and limitations.

- **Shared Values:** Focus on your shared values and goals as parents.

Navigating the postpartum period and parenthood with POTS is challenging, but it is possible. By prioritizing your health, building sustainable routines, and utilizing your support system, you can thrive in your new normal.

Navigating the New Normal

- **Expect Gradual Recovery:** Long-term recovery is variable and takes time. Be patient and realistic.

- **Master Pacing:** Use energy conservation strategies to manage the demands of newborn care and avoid the boom-bust cycle.

- **Rebuild Strength:** Gradually recondition your body with POTS-friendly exercises and prioritize pelvic floor rehabilitation.

- **Prioritize Mental Health:** Monitor for PMADs and seek ongoing support for your mental well-being.

- **Nurture Your Relationship:** Maintain open communication and adjust roles and expectations with your partner.

Chapter 11: Templates and Checklists, and Resources

This section provides practical tools to help you manage your pregnancy and postpartum journey. Use these templates and checklists to organize your information, communicate effectively with your medical team, and track your progress.

POTS-Specific Birth Plan Template (Vaginal and Cesarean considerations)

POTS-Specific Birth Plan

Patient Name: [Your Name]

Date of Birth: [Your DOB]

Medical Record Number: [Your MRN]

Emergency Contact: [Name and Phone Number]

Diagnosis: Postural Orthostatic Tachycardia Syndrome (POTS) / Dysautonomia.

Key Information: POTS is an autonomic nervous system disorder that causes rapid heart rate (tachycardia), dizziness, and blood pressure instability, especially when upright. I am at high risk for sudden drops in blood pressure (hypotension).

General Management:

- **Triggers:** My symptoms are worsened by heat, prolonged standing, and dehydration.

- **Room Temperature:** Please keep the room cool.

- **Mobility:** I need assistance when getting out of bed or walking to prevent falls.

Hydration:

- **IV Fluids:** Please establish IV access and start continuous IV fluids (Normal Saline or Lactated Ringers) immediately upon admission. Maintaining blood volume is critical.

Monitoring:

- **Vital Signs:** Continuous monitoring of heart rate and frequent blood pressure checks are necessary.

- **Fetal Monitoring:** Continuous electronic fetal monitoring is expected.

Positioning:

- **Avoid Supine Position:** I cannot lie flat on my back. This causes supine hypotension syndrome.

- **Left Uterine Displacement:** Please ensure I am tilted to the side (left uterine displacement) during monitoring, procedures, and delivery.

- **Preferred Positions:** Side-lying is often the most stable position for me.

Anesthesia (Epidural/Spinal):

- **Anesthesia Consult:** Please refer to the anesthesia consultation note in my chart.

- **High Risk of Hypotension:** Epidurals and spinal blocks can cause severe hypotension.

- **Fluid Pre-loading:** I need aggressive IV fluid pre-loading (1-2 liters) before anesthesia administration.

- **Vasopressors:** Please have vasopressors (e.g., phenylephrine) readily available to treat hypotension promptly.

Labor and Delivery:

- **Pushing:** I may need assistance with pushing due to fatigue or dizziness. Side-lying pushing is preferred.

- **Minimize Exertion:** Please minimize unnecessary exertion and prolonged standing.

Postpartum:

- **Compression:** I will wear an abdominal binder and compression stockings immediately after delivery.

- **Mobility:** I need assistance with mobilization to prevent falls.

- **Hydration:** Please continue IV fluids postpartum as needed, and encourage oral hydration.

Medications:

- **Current Medications:** [List your current medications and dosages]

- **Medication Plan:** [Describe the plan for taking your medications during labor and postpartum]

Thank you for your cooperation and support in ensuring a safe delivery.

Medical provider communication scripts and advocacy starters

Introducing POTS to a New Provider:

"I have Postural Orthostatic Tachycardia Syndrome, or POTS. It's an autonomic nervous system disorder that affects my heart rate and blood pressure regulation. The main symptoms I experience are [list your main symptoms]. I am sharing this information to ensure I receive safe and appropriate care."

Requesting Accommodations (e.g., IV Fluids):

"Due to my POTS, I am very sensitive to dehydration, which can cause severe symptoms and instability. My specialist recommends aggressive IV hydration during labor. Can we ensure that IV fluids are started immediately upon admission?"

Addressing Dismissal or Misunderstanding:

"I understand that fatigue/dizziness is common in pregnancy, but what I am experiencing is severe and consistent with my POTS diagnosis. Can we discuss strategies to manage this medically?"

"I appreciate your perspective, but my symptoms are physiological, not psychological. I need us to focus on the medical management of my POTS."

Asking Clarifying Questions:

"Can you explain the reasoning behind that recommendation? I want to make sure I understand the risks and benefits."

"What are the alternatives to this approach? Are there options that might be better tolerated with my condition?"

During Procedures (e.g., Ultrasound):

"I cannot lie flat on my back due to supine hypotension syndrome. Can we use a wedge to tilt me to the side, or can I be positioned on an incline?"

"I am starting to feel dizzy/nauseous. I need to shift to my side immediately."

Daily symptom, hydration, and electrolyte logs

Daily Log Template

Date:

Weight (if tracking):

Hydration:

- Total Fluid Intake (Liters/Ounces):

- Electrolyte Intake (Grams of Sodium/Type of Electrolyte):

Medications:

- [Medication Name]: [Dose], [Time]

- [Medication Name]: [Dose], [Time]

Compression:

- Type (Waist-high/Thigh-high/Abdominal Binder):

- Hours Worn:

Activity/Exercise:

- Type of Activity:

- Duration:

- Intensity/Heart Rate:

Symptoms (Rate 1-10, 1=mild, 10=severe):

- Dizziness/Lightheadedness:

- Tachycardia/Palpitations:

- Fatigue:

- Brain Fog:

- Nausea/Vomiting:

- Shortness of Breath:

- Pain (e.g., Headache, Joint Pain):

Notes/Triggers:

(e.g., Poor sleep, heat exposure, stress, specific foods)

Medication tracking sheets

(Similar to the medication section in the Daily Log, but focused specifically on tracking medication adherence, side effects, and effectiveness over time).

POTS-Specific Hospital Go-Bag Checklist

POTS Essentials:

- [ ] Electrolyte powders or tablets (your preferred brand)
- [ ] Salty snacks (pretzels, nuts, crackers)
- [ ] Large water bottle with a straw
- [ ] Compression stockings (waist-high or thigh-high)
- [ ] Abdominal binder (for postpartum use)
- [ ] Portable fan (battery-operated or USB)
- [ ] Cooling towel
- [ ] Eye mask and earplugs (to reduce sensory overload)

Medical Information:

- [ ] Multiple copies of your POTS-Specific Birth Plan
- [ ] Medical summary letter from your specialist
- [ ] Current medication list and allergies
- [ ] Insurance information and ID

Comfort Items:

- [ ] Comfortable pajamas or gown (button-down for breastfeeding)
- [ ] Robe
- [ ] Slippers or non-slip socks
- [ ] Toiletries (including lip balm and moisturizer)
- [ ] Phone and charger (extra-long cord)
- [ ] Pillow (hospitals pillows are often uncomfortable)

Baby Items:

- [ ] Going-home outfit
- [ ] Car seat (installed in the car)
- [ ] Swaddle or blanket

Emergency contact lists and Medical Summary Template

Medical Summary Template

Name: [Your Name]

Date of Birth: [Your DOB]

Diagnoses:

- Postural Orthostatic Tachycardia Syndrome (POTS) - [Type if known, e.g., Hyperadrenergic, Hypovolemic]
- [Comorbidities, e.g., Ehlers-Danlos Syndrome (hEDS), Mast Cell Activation Syndrome (MCAS), Migraine]

Allergies/Sensitivities:

- [List any allergies to medications, foods, or materials]

Current Medications:

- [Medication Name]: [Dose], [Frequency]
- [Medication Name]: [Dose], [Frequency]

Baseline Vital Signs:

- Resting Heart Rate:
- Blood Pressure Range:

POTS Symptoms and Management:

- Main Symptoms: [List your main symptoms]
- Triggers: [List your main triggers]
- Management Strategies: [e.g., High salt/fluid intake, compression, medications]

Emergency Protocol:

- If found unconscious or severely symptomatic:
    - Check airway, breathing, circulation.
    - Administer IV fluids (Normal Saline) if available.
    - Monitor vital signs closely.
    - Transport to [Preferred Hospital].

Medical Providers:

- **POTS Specialist:** [Name, Specialty, Phone Number]
- **MFM/OB:** [Name, Phone Number]
- **Primary Care Physician:** [Name, Phone Number]
- **Other Specialists:** [Name, Specialty, Phone Number]

Emergency Contacts:

- **Primary Contact:** [Name, Relationship, Phone Number]

- **Secondary Contact:** [Name, Relationship, Phone Number]

Postpartum Support Plan and Organizer

Postpartum Support Plan

Goal: Prioritize maternal recovery and bonding with the baby.

Key Principles: Rest, hydration, pacing, and asking for help.

Support Team:

- **Partner:** [Name]

- **Family:** [Name(s)]

- **Friends:** [Name(s)]

- **Hired Help (if applicable):** [e.g., Postpartum Doula, Cleaning Service]

Division of Responsibilities (Weeks 1-6):

- **Newborn Care (Feedings, Changing, Soothing):**
  - Daytime: [Who is responsible]
  - Nighttime: [Who is responsible - specify shifts]

- **Household Tasks:**
  - Cooking/Meals: [Who is responsible/Meal Train organizer]
  - Cleaning: [Who is responsible]
  - Laundry: [Who is responsible]
  - Grocery Shopping/Errands: [Who is responsible]

- **Maternal Care (Ensuring Mom rests, hydrates, eats):**
  - [Who is responsible]

Rest Plan:

- **Napping Strategy:** [e.g., Nap when baby sleeps, scheduled naps]

- **Sleep Strategy:** [e.g., Sleep shifts, uninterrupted sleep periods]

Visitor Policy:

- [e.g., Limited visitors, short visits, visitors must be healthy and helpful]

Self-Care Plan:

- **Hydration Goal:** [e.g., 3-4 Liters/day]

- **Nutrition Goal:** [e.g., 3 meals + snacks/day]

- **Compression:** [e.g., Wear daily]

- **Mental Health:** [e.g., Therapy appointments, support group check-ins]

Emergency Contacts:

- **MFM/OB:** [Phone Number]

- **POTS Specialist:** [Phone Number]

- **Mental Health Professional:** [Phone Number]

- **Lactation Consultant:** [Phone Number]

Glossary of Terms

- **Autonomic Nervous System (ANS):** The part of the nervous system that controls involuntary bodily functions, such as heart rate, blood pressure, digestion, and temperature regulation.

- **Blood Volume:** The total amount of blood circulating in the body. Low blood volume (hypovolemia) is common in POTS.

- **Compression Garments:** Tight-fitting clothing (stockings, abdominal binders) that provide external pressure to prevent blood pooling and improve circulation.

- **Deconditioning:** The loss of muscle mass and cardiovascular fitness due to inactivity or immobility. Deconditioning worsens POTS symptoms.

- **Dysautonomia:** A general term for disorders of the autonomic nervous system. POTS is a form of dysautonomia.

- **Ehlers-Danlos Syndrome (EDS):** A group of genetic connective tissue disorders characterized by joint hypermobility and tissue fragility. Often co-occurs with POTS.

- **Hemodynamics:** The study of blood flow and circulation.

- **Hyperadrenergic POTS:** A subtype of POTS characterized by an overactive sympathetic nervous system (high levels of adrenaline/norepinephrine).

- **Hyperemesis Gravidarum (HG):** Extreme, persistent nausea and vomiting during pregnancy leading to dehydration and weight loss.

- **Hypotension:** Low blood pressure.

- **Hypovolemia:** Low blood volume.

- **Mast Cell Activation Syndrome (MCAS):** A condition where mast cells inappropriately release chemicals (like histamine), causing allergic-type symptoms and inflammation. Often co-occurs with POTS.

- **Maternal-Fetal Medicine (MFM):** A specialist in high-risk obstetrics.

- **Orthostatic Intolerance:** The inability to tolerate being upright, resulting in symptoms like dizziness, tachycardia, and fatigue.

- **Pacing:** A strategy for managing chronic illness by balancing activity with rest to avoid symptom flares and the "boom-bust" cycle.

- **Postural Orthostatic Tachycardia Syndrome (POTS):** A disorder characterized by a significant increase in heart rate upon standing, accompanied by symptoms of orthostatic intolerance.

- **Pre-syncope:** The feeling that you are about to faint.

- **Supine Hypotension Syndrome:** A condition in late pregnancy where the uterus compresses the vena cava when lying flat on the back, causing a drop in blood pressure.

- **Syncope:** Fainting.

- **Tachycardia:** Rapid heart rate (over 100 bpm at rest).

- **Vasodilation:** Widening of blood vessels.

- **Vasoconstriction:** Tightening of blood vessels.

- **Venous Pooling:** The accumulation of blood in the lower body due to gravity and inadequate vasoconstriction.

Summary of Latest Clinical Evidence and Recommendations

(This section would provide a concise summary of the key findings and recommendations from the latest research and clinical guidelines on POTS and pregnancy, referencing the studies cited throughout the book).

References

Bourne, K. M., Sheldon, R. S., & Raj, S. R. (2021). Compression garments for the treatment of orthostatic hypotension. *Cochrane Database of Systematic Reviews*, (2).

Dangel, A., Vasanth, S., & Stiles, L. E. (2023). Symptoms of postural orthostatic tachycardia syndrome in pregnancy: a cross-sectional, community-based survey. *The Journal of Maternal-Fetal & Neonatal Medicine*, *36*(2).
https://doi.org/10.1080/14767058.2023.2236129

D'Oria, V., Varlotta, S., & Mastroianni, C. (2023). Hyperemesis Gravidarum and Postural Orthostatic Tachycardia Syndrome (POTS): A Case Report and Review of the Literature. *Journal of Clinical Medicine*, *12*(5), 1835.
https://doi.org/10.3390/jcm12051835

Dysautonomia International. (n.d.). *Instructions for POTS Exercise Program—Children's Hospital of Philadelphia*. Retrieved August 17, 2025, from
https://www.dysautonomiainternational.org/pdf/CHOP_Modified_Dallas_POTS_Exercise_Program.pdf

Fu, Q., & Levine, B. D. (2018). Exercise and non-pharmacological treatment of POTS. *Autonomic Neuroscience: Basic and Clinical*, *215*, 20–27. https://doi.org/10.1016/j.autneu.2018.07.001

Kanjwal, K., Jaradeh, S., & Grubb, B. P. (2009). Outcomes of pregnancy in patients with preexisting postural tachycardia syndrome. *Pacing and Clinical Electrophysiology*, *32*(8), 1000–1003.
https://doi.org/10.1111/j.1540-8159.2009.02420.x

LactMed. (n.d.). Drugs and Lactation Database. National Library of Medicine. Retrieved August 17, 2025, from https://www.ncbi.nlm.nih.gov/books/NBK501922/

Morgan, K., Ramirez, N., & Blitshteyn, S. (2022). POTS and Pregnancy: A Review of Literature and Recommendations for Evaluation and Treatment. *International Journal of Women's Health*, *14*, 1831–1847. https://doi.org/10.2147/IJWH.S366667

POTS UK. (2021). *Postural Tachycardia Syndrome and Pregnancy*. https://www.potsuk.org/wp-content/uploads/2021/10/Postural_Tachycardia_Syndrome_and_P regnancy_Leaflet_Feb_2021.pdf

Raj, S. R., Fedorowski, A., & Sheldon, R. S. (2022). Postural orthostatic tachycardia syndrome: definitions and diagnosis. *Journal of the American College of Cardiology*, *79*(18), 1813-1827.

Sanghavi, M., & Rutherford, J. D. (2014). Cardiovascular physiology of pregnancy. *Circulation*, *130*(12), 1003–1008. https://doi.org/10.1161/CIRCULATIONAHA.114.009029

Vernino, S., Bourne, K. M., Stiles, L. E., Grubb, B. P., Fedorowski, A., Stewart, J. M., Arnold, A. C., Pace, L. A., Axelsson, J., Boris, J. R., Moak, J. P., Goodman, B. P., Chémali, K. R., Chung, T. H., Goldstein, D. S., Diedrich, A., Miglis, M. G., Cortez, M. M., Miller, A. J., ... Raj, S. R. (2021). Postural orthostatic tachycardia syndrome (POTS): State of the science and clinical care from a 2019 National Institutes of Health Expert Consensus Meeting - Part 1. *Autonomic Neuroscience: Basic and Clinical*, *235*, 102828. https://doi.org/10.1016/j.autneu.2021.102828

Zha, K., Brook, J., & Blitshteyn, S. (2022). Gluten-free diet in postural orthostatic tachycardia syndrome (POTS). *Autonomic Neuroscience*, *237*, 102902. https://doi.org/10.1016/j.autneu.2021.102902